THE COMPLETE GUIDE TO
PREGNANCY AND FITNESS

THE COMPLETE GUIDE TO
PREGNANCY AND FITNESS

Morc Coulson and Sarah Bolitho

BLOOMSBURY

LONDON · NEW DELHI · NEW YORK · SYDNEY

Published by Bloomsbury Publishing Plc
50 Bedford Square
London WC1B 3DP
www.bloomsbury.com

ISBN (print): 978 1 4081 5381 9
ISBN (epub): 978 1 4081 7875 1
ISBN (epdf): 978 1 4081 7876 8

Acknowledgements
Cover photograph © Shutterstock. All inside photographs © Grant Pritchard with the exception of the following: p.viii, p.122 © Getty Images; p.58, p.86 © Shutterstock
Illustrations by David Gardner
Designed by James Watson
Commissioned by Charlotte Croft
Edited by Sarah Cole

This book is produced using paper that is made from wood grown in managed, sustainable forests. It is natural, renewable and recyclable. The logging and manufacturing processes conform to the environmental regulations of the country of origin.

Typeset in 10.75pt on 14pt Adobe Caslon by seagulls.net

Printed and bound in China by C&C Offset Printing Co

10 9 8 7 6 5 4 3 2 1

CONTENTS

To my lovely kids, Jackson, Maddison, Ashleigh and Nicholas who just go to show that pregnancy is all worthwhile; and to my lovely wife Lorretta who actually had to go through it! Love you all,

Morc

This is dedicated to my three fantastic children, Lucie, Danny and James, each of whom made the experience of pregnancy worth every symptom and who are now three of the best people I know. This is also for my granddaughter Isla, who enabled me to experience pregnancy from a slight distance while my daughter went through it!

Thanks also goes to all at Crown Fitness, Pontypridd, for allowing us to use their facilities for the photo shoot, as well as to Sam Thomas and Sarah Dowson who are the models in the photographs. Both were 38 weeks pregnant at the time and have now given birth to healthy boys, Elis and Oliver.

Sarah

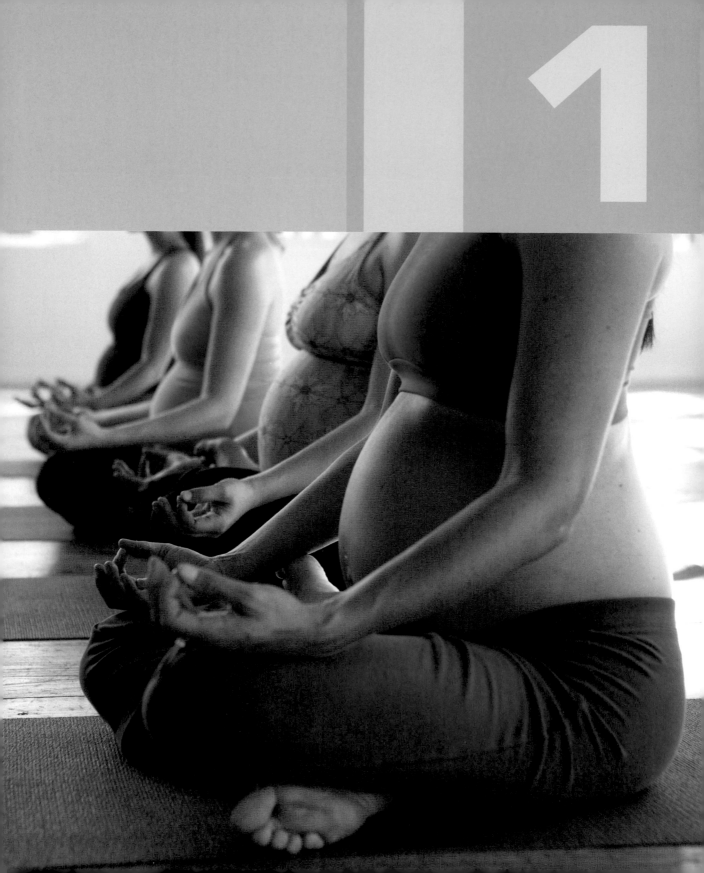

PART ONE

UNDERPINNING KNOWLEDGE

INTRODUCTION // TO PREGNANCY

KEY POINTS

- Instructors wishing to prescribe exercise programmes to women in this population should hold a current Level 2 Fitness Instructor qualification in Gym or Exercise to Music as validated by the Register of Exercise Professionals, as well as a current recognised qualification in ante- and postnatal exercise.
- Skills Active is the overseeing body responsible for instructor qualifications in line with the Qualifications and Curriculum Framework (QCF) for health and fitness.
- Pregnancy can be split roughly into three time periods, each lasting approximately three months, which are known as 'trimesters'. The first trimester is usually cited as being 0–13 weeks, the second trimester is 14–27 weeks and the third trimester is 28–42 weeks.
- The period up to 6 weeks after birth is known as the immediate postnatal period and the period from then up to about a year afterwards is referred to as the extended postnatal period.
- A 'normal' pregnancy duration is referred to in medical terms as being 40 weeks plus or minus 2 or 3 weeks, however any baby that is born between 37 and 42 weeks is considered to be 'full term'.
- Babies have been known to survive delivery as early as only 22 weeks into the pregnancy even though survival rates can be low.
- It is possible to estimate the due date or 'expected delivery date' (EDD) as it is also known, if the pregnancy is of the normal duration.

PREGNANCY AND FITNESS

Within the health and fitness environment pregnant women are categorised as a 'special population' as they have particular needs over and above those of the general 'apparently healthy' population. For this reason, those women who are within this population should have a minimum understanding of the condition in order to make informed decisions regarding exercise related to their condition. It is also advisable to seek guidance from a suitably qualified person prior to undertaking any form of exercise programme.

Within the National Qualifications Framework (NQF) for health and fitness, those instructors wishing to prescribe exercise programmes to women in this population should hold a current Level 2 qualification as validated by the Register of Exercise Professionals (REPs) as well as a current recognised qualification in ante- and postnatal exercise. The current Level 2 Award in Fitness Instructing includes limited information for instructors whose participants or clients become pregnant or who occasionally get pregnant women attending their classes. However, while this information gives the instructor enough information to ensure that any class or session is safe for an experienced exerciser who becomes pregnant, it is not sufficient to work with this client group on a regular basis or to work with previously inactive women who are pregnant.

It is not the purpose of this book to discuss reproduction or the progression of pregnancy in 'clinical' detail, but to consider the implications that pregnancy has for exercise and activity. If the reader requires further information on these aspects of pregnancy there are numerous books available that cover the topic in great detail.

Pregnancy can be split roughly into three-month time periods, which are better known as 'trimesters' as seen in figure 1.1. Once the mother has given birth there are two further time periods

For more information relating to qualifications within the industry please refer to www.skillsactive.com and for information relating to the professional qualifications register please refer to www.exerciseregister.org. The content of this book is aligned to Level 3 National Occupational Standards for Ante- and Postnatal Exercise and is an ideal accompaniment to the courses available from leading training providers.

known as the immediate postnatal period and the extended postnatal period.

The three-trimester period prior to birth is referred to as the 'antenatal' period, whereas when a woman has given birth, the period up to about a year afterwards is known as the 'postnatal' period. A 'normal' pregnancy (one which is considered to be of a standard duration) is referred to in medical terms as being 40 weeks plus or minus 2 or 3 weeks. In other words, a normal pregnancy lasts for a duration of between 38 and 42 weeks. It is possible to estimate the due date or 'expected delivery date' (EDD), as it is otherwise known, if the pregnancy is of the normal duration. The following steps show an example of how to estimate the EDD.

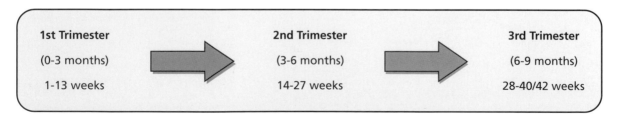

Figure 1.1 Approximate duration of antenatal and postnatal periods. Note: The time frames used are those suggested by the American College of Obstetricians & Gynecologists (ACOG)

- *Step 1:* Write down the date of last menstrual period (LMP), e.g. 1 February 2011
- *Step 2:* Add on seven days = 8 February 2011
- *Step 3:* Add on nine calendar months to get the EDD = 8 November 2011.

In clinical or medical terms, any baby that is born between 37 and 42 weeks is considered to be 'full term'. In other words, it is assumed that the baby has reached its full development potential. However, this does not mean that babies born outside of this period would necessarily not reach full development potential. Due to the many advances in medical technology that have taken place over the past few decades, babies have been known to survive delivery as early as only 22 weeks into the pregnancy (which is known as 'premature birth'). Unfortunately, the survival rate of a baby is only about 1 per cent when born at 22 weeks, but increases to around 17 per cent by 23 weeks and to around 80 per cent by 28 weeks. That said, for most women once the pregnancy is established they can look forward to a happy arrival in approximately 40 weeks.

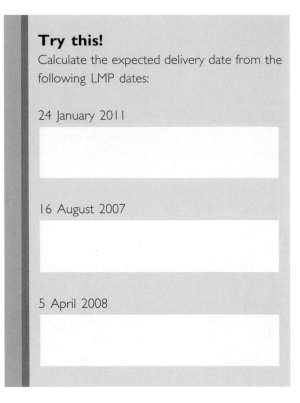

Try this!
Calculate the expected delivery date from the following LMP dates:

24 January 2011

16 August 2007

5 April 2008

COMMON SYMPTOMS OF PREGNANCY

2

KEY POINTS

- There is a wide range of both physiological and psychological symptoms that are associated with the state of pregnancy.
- Physiological symptoms are to do with the body and psychological symptoms are to do with the mind.
- Most symptoms of pregnancy can be uncomfortable but they are generally a sign of healthy pregnancy.
- Some of the common symptoms are not always present during pregnancy and are not always consistent.
- There are some symptoms that are only common to particular trimesters however some symptoms can persist throughout the entire duration of the pregnancy.
- About one in eight pregnancies end in an early miscarriage before the pregnancy is actually detected.
- Some symptoms can be a sign of a very serious complication of pregnancy such as sudden swelling/ oedema which is a sign of 'pregnancy-induced hypertension' (PIH) or pre-eclampsia, and if left untreated or not reported, it can be potentially fatal for mother and baby.

PHYSIOLOGICAL AND PSYCHOLOGICAL SYMPTOMS

There are many symptoms that are associated with the state of pregnancy. There are those known as 'physiological' symptoms, which are to do with the body and those known as 'psychological' symptoms, which are to do with the mind. Unfortunately, for mothers-to-be most of these symptoms are often uncomfortable and difficult to manage. However on a positive note, they are generally considered to be an indication of a healthy pregnancy.

Not all of the common symptoms experienced by mothers-to-be are always present during the course of a pregnancy and they are not always consistent in nature. Generally speaking, however, there are a number of common symptoms occurring within each trimester, which are summarised in table 2.1 (these symptoms will be expanded on throughout the course of this book). The instructor should note that some of the symptoms can be present in all trimesters.

Table 2.1	Common symptoms associated with trimesters	
First trimester	**Second trimester**	**Third trimester**
Nausea and sickness often occur.	The linea nigra develops (dark vertical line on the abdomen) as the abdomen continues to expand.	The woman can become tired very easily.
Tiredness and breathlessness occur with any increases in activity.	Hormones tend to stabilise during this period and mood improves.	Discomfort is often felt at this later stage.
There is an increase in resting heart rate (of about 5–10bpm) and breathing rate, which in turn increases the metabolic rate.	The intestinal tract relaxes.	Posture continues to be a problem and can exacerbate existing problems.
The woman undergoes hormonal changes such as the release of relaxin, which allows ligaments to stretch.	Colostrum secretion occurs from the breasts.	Some women develop high blood pressure and fluid retention.
There is a risk of miscarriage around weeks 8–12.	The woman can suffer bleeding gums.	Braxton Hicks contractions can occur. These are uterine contractions that occur throughout pregnancy but are not usually felt until later on when they may be mistaken for labour contractions.
The breasts and the uterus tend to enlarge.	Backache is common due to certain postural changes.	The woman can become anxious and not sleep well.
Women gain on average about 1–3kg.	Weight gain on average is about 6–8kg.	Weight gain on average is about 3–4kg.
		Venous return (blood flow back to the heart) can be reduced, causing breathlessness.
		Increased urination can occur.

FIRST TRIMESTER – WEEKS 0–13
Nausea and sickness

This is often one of the more common initial indicators of pregnancy. It is thought to be due mainly to the presence of the hormone known as 'human chorionic gonadotropin' (HCG) but it could also be a result of the mother-to-be having low blood sugar levels.

Tiredness

Mothers-to-be can become tired and fatigued very quickly and very often. This is particularly due to the changes in the blood chemistry, resulting in a reduced oxygen-carrying capacity, and can also be due to low blood sugar levels. This cumulative effect can be quite pronounced in those who are not particularly fit prior to conception.

Breathlessness

The area of the brain (beyond the scope of this book) that is responsible for the control of breathing becomes more sensitive to carbon dioxide during pregnancy. It will speed up breathing sooner than usual during activity, causing breathlessness even at very low levels of activity. It is recommended therefore that fitness levels are increased prior to conception to help minimise this effect as much as possible.

Mood changes

Not all women suffer this particular effect but those who are not used to changes in hormone levels (first time pregnant women, for instance) may find themselves dealing with emotional swings that can range from mild to severe and may be sudden in onset.

Sensory changes

Many women experience an altered sensitivity to taste and smell throughout pregnancy, particularly in the first trimester. Mothers-to-be can also acquire unusual tastes or cravings, including the condition 'pica' where non-food substances such as coal or paper are eaten.

Risk of miscarriage

According to many sources of statistics, there tends to be a higher risk of miscarriage or spontaneous abortion in the first trimester (more commonly between weeks 8–12 and around the time the period would have occurred) than there is in the other two trimesters. Also, around weeks 8–12, all of the organ systems of the embryo, which is now referred to as a 'foetus', should be in place and the placenta should be developing. If however, there are significant defects in the embryo or there are problems with the placenta, then the pregnancy may naturally terminate at this point. It is stated that as many as one in eight pregnancies end in an early miscarriage before the pregnancy is actually detected. By 12 weeks, if the foetal heartbeat or the ultrasound scan is normal, miscarriage risk drops to about 1 per cent.

Joint instability

Due to the influence of the hormone relaxin, which increases in level during pregnancy, connective tissue within ligaments and tendons starts to become more elastic (see page 16). This in turn will make joints less stable.

Breast tenderness

Breasts may become swollen and very sore and sensitive due to hormonal changes in preparation for the production of mother's milk.

Weight gain

Pregnant women often gain weight at this stage as the body is storing fat in order to deal with feeding the baby over the long-term duration of the pregnancy. However, a relatively small gain of between 1 and 3kg is considered healthy at this stage.

SECOND TRIMESTER – WEEKS 14–27
Pregnancy starts to show

The foetus continues to grow and the uterus expands up and out of the pelvis and into the abdomen. At about 20 weeks, or earlier in a second or successive pregnancy, the uterus has normally risen up to the level of the navel.

Decrease in nausea and sickness

As the pregnancy becomes fully established, sickness should decrease and appetite and mood should improve as the hormones tend to stabilise. This happens because the placenta is fully developed and has taken over the production of the pregnancy hormones. It should be noted, however, that for some mothers nausea and even sickness may continue into the second trimester and beyond.

Posture

There is a forward shift in centre of gravity of the mother-to-be due to the uterus moving up and out of the pelvis, which can affect posture. The main effect tends to be an increase in lumbar lordosis (a curved lower back), which can cause considerable back pain.

Weight gain

The main weight gain (see page 24/25 for a breakdown of the distribution of weight gain) occurs in this trimester as the foetus gains in size. This is commonly in the region of 6–8kg.

Joint stability

The hormone relaxin continues to affect the stability of the joints, particularly in the region of the pelvis and lower back, as described in the first trimester.

Breast fluid leakage

The breasts may start to leak a fluid known as 'colostrum' (or 'first milk') in this trimester, however this mainly occurs later in the third trimester.

THIRD TRIMESTER – WEEKS 28–42
Fatigue

The extra weight of the baby and any maternal weight gain causes increased tiredness as the mother-to-be is carrying several kilograms above her normal weight.

Discomfort

By this stage the expanding uterus and the baby will extend to the top of the abdominal cavity and up towards the breast bone. Some internal organs are likely to be compressed as a result of this, which can lead to obvious discomfort for the mother-to-be.

Posture

There is likely to be a greater forward shift of centre of gravity which again increases lordosis (curved lower back) and can contribute to kyphosis (rounded shoulders).

Fluid retention (oedema)

Due to the many hormonal influences, fluid may be retained in the tissues, particularly around the wrists, hands and ankles, causing swelling which is known as 'oedema'. Note: Sudden swelling/ oedema can be a sign of two very serious complications of pregnancy, pregnancy-induced hypertension (PIH) or pre-eclampsia. If left untreated or not reported, either condition can be potentially fatal for mother and baby.

Breathlessness

Sensitivity to carbon dioxide (partially responsible for breathing rate) further increases and with the pressure of the growing uterus on the lungs, can result in increased breathlessness for the mother-to-be.

Increased urination (peeing)

The pressure of the baby and the uterus on the bladder increases the frequency and urgency of urination. This is also known by the term 'micturition'.

Breast leakage

It is in this trimester that the woman's breasts more commonly leak colostrum or 'first milk' as the mother-to-be prepares for lactation (feeding the baby).

IMMEDIATE POSTNATAL PERIOD – 0–6 WEEKS

Extreme fatigue

Due to the physiological and psychological demands of a new baby (in particular regular feeding throughout the night) the mother is likely to be feeling exhausted.

Breasts

Lactating breasts may be heavy and leak milk. They may also be sore or chafed as a result of the baby regularly feeding. This may lead to infection, called mastitis, which can be very painful.

Postnatal bleeding (lochia)

Bleeding from the site of the placenta may continue after the birth of the baby for a period of up to 3 weeks or more. This can in some cases be quite heavy and may be accompanied by moderate to severe cramps in the early postnatal weeks which can be uncomfortable and cause some anxiety about leaking.

Joint instability

The effect of the hormone relaxin on joints (see page 16) continues after delivery and can last for up to nine months postnatally, particularly in second and subsequent or multiple pregnancies. Exercise advice should be sought for this extended period.

Diastasis recti

The abdominal muscles which have been lengthened around the growing uterus can in some cases split or separate during pregnancy (see page 27), which has an effect on the type of exercises that must be avoided in this period.

EXTENDED POSTNATAL PERIOD – 6 WEEKS PLUS

Most women will have a 6-week postnatal check-up with their midwife (this is always encouraged) and, if given the all clear to return to normal activities, she can generally start or return to an appropriate level of exercise and activity as prescribed by a suitably qualified person.

PHYSIOLOGICAL CHANGES IN PREGNANCY

// **3**

KEY POINTS

- The physiological changes in the body during pregnancy can be grouped into several areas such as hormonal, thermoregulation, cardiovascular, respiratory, metabolic, gastrointestinal and postural changes.
- Hormonal changes include the release of relaxin, oestrogen and progesterone.
- Thermoregulation changes include mother's core temperature going up, causing the pregnant 'glow', increase in heat loss and quicker sweating.
- Cardiovascular changes include a blood volume increase, red blood cell mass increase, blood vessel wall dilation, resting heart rate rise, cardiac output increase, the left ventricle enlargement and increased blood flow to the skin.
- Respiratory changes can include increased ventilation rate and depth, the brain being more sensitive to levels of carbon dioxide, decreased residual volume, increased oxygen consumption and hyperventilation.
- Metabolic adaptations include resting metabolic rate increase, symptoms of mild diabetes, carbohydrate energy supplies preferentially used by the foetus and a dip in maternal blood sugar levels.
- Gastrointestinal changes include relaxation of smooth muscle tissue.
- Postural and musculoskeletal changes include centre of gravity disturbance, diastasis recti and ligament relaxation.
- Other effects as a result of changes during pregnancy include carpal tunnel syndrome (CTS), chloasma (dark pigmentation on the face), leg cramps, stretch marks, hyperemesis gravidarum (excessive vomiting) and either hair loss or an increase in hair growth.

AREAS OF PHYSIOLOGICAL CHANGE

There are many changes to the mother-to-be that take place in the early stages of a pregnancy which can cause the common symptoms as discussed in the previous chapter. These changes can be classified as either physiological or psychological, for which there is a substantial amount of

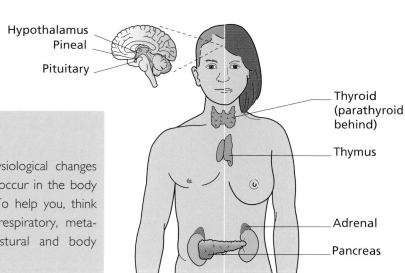

Hypothalamus
Pineal
Pituitary

Thyroid
(parathyroid
behind)

Thymus

Adrenal

Pancreas

Ovaries

Testes

Figure 3.1 Glands of the endocrine system

research-based evidence relating to the changes within each classification. Rather than be thought of as problematic, these changes are essential for a variety of different reasons. The main reason is arguably to make sure that a constant supply of energy to the foetus and mother-to-be is always available.

In terms of the physiological changes, there are many effects that take place throughout the duration of the pregnancy and into the post-natal period.

The physiological changes that occur within the body can be further divided into several subclassifications such as hormonal, thermoregulation, cardiovascular, respiratory, metabolic, gastrointestinal and postural changes. Table 3.1 lists and gives a brief description of what might be considered to be the main changes that usually occur.

HORMONAL CHANGES
There is a type of chemical messenger system within the body, known as the 'endocrine' system, which is capable of sending messages by using hormones (*hormon* means 'to excite'). These hormones are secreted by glands which are situated around the body. Most hormones are circulated via the bloodstream and therefore this system can be quite slow compared to the nervous system, which is an immediate system as it uses electrical impulses.

The main endocrine glands in the body include the pineal, pituitary, thyroid, parathyroid and adrenal glands. There are other tissues that secrete hormones such as the hypothalamus, pancreas, thymus, ovaries, testes, kidneys and stomach, but these are generally not referred to as endocrine glands. Figure 3.1 shows where the endocrine glands are situated.

Table 3.1	Typical physiological changes associated with pregnancy	
Type of change/ adaptation	**Changes occurring**	**Description**
Hormonal	Relaxin release	This is released from the ovaries up to about 12–14 weeks when it is then released from the placenta. It can loosen ligaments postnatally for up to six months.
	Oestrogen release	The levels tend to remain high throughout pregnancy as it promotes foetal growth, causes breast enlargement and stimulates colostrum production.
	Progesterone release	The levels are high throughout pregnancy as it relaxes smooth muscle, stabilises blood pressure and stimulates colostrum. Greater insulin sensitivity to glucose can occur due to hormone level increase.
Thermoregulation	Mother's core temperature goes up	Temperature can increase by 0.6°C at the start and remain elevated for about 20 weeks.
	Pregnant glow	Some areas of skin become hotter by up to 2–6°C.
	Increase in heat loss	In early pregnancy heat dissipation is increased by up to 30% and in late pregnancy by up to 70% due to increased body mass.
	Quicker sweating	The blood flow to skin increases and the breathing rate elevates, both increasing heat loss.
Cardiovascular	Blood volume increases	The volume of blood in the body can increase by as much as 50% to help supply oxygen to the foetus.
	Red blood cell mass increases	Red blood cells can also increase by as much as 20–30% in order to supply oxygen to the foetus.
	Blood vessel walls dilate	The size of the blood vessels increase to allow greater blood flow, which results in not enough circulating volume of blood to maintain blood pressure, known as vascular underfill.
	Resting heart rate (RHR) rises	RHR can rise by as much as 10–15bpm.
	Cardiac output increases	The amount of blood pumped out of the heart every minute can increase by about 30%.
	The left ventricle enlarges	The chamber in the heart that pumps blood to the body can enlarge by about 20%.
	Blood flow to the skin increases	This occurs to help cool the body.

Respiratory	Increased ventilation rate and depth	This just means that breathing increases and the amount of air taken in and out (tidal volume) increases by about 40–50%.
	The brain is more sensitive to levels of carbon dioxide	This can be common at about 12 weeks due to the release of the hormone progesterone.
	Decreased residual volume	This is partly responsible for the increase in breathing rate.
	Increased oxygen consumption	The amount of 'spare' space in the lungs decreases.
	Hyperventilation can occur	The amount of oxygen that is used up from the air increases by up to about 30%.
Metabolic	Resting metabolic rate increases	The amount of energy used in the body at rest can increase by up to 20%.
	Symptoms of mild diabetes	This is due to a delayed insulin response.
	Carbohydrate energy supplies are preferentially used by foetus	There is a high usage (in percentage terms compared to normal) of carbohydrate by the foetus so this should be taken into account by the mother especially when exercising.
	Maternal blood sugar levels dip	This happens about every 6–8 hours due to the usage by the foetus.
Gastrointestinal	Relaxation of smooth muscle tissue	Progesterone relaxes smooth muscle tissue which can lead to slower digestion and increased incidence of constipation, haemorrhoids (piles) and indigestion. Acid reflux can also occur which can lead to vomiting and dehydration.
Postural and musculoskeletal	Centre of gravity disturbance	During the growth of the baby the centre of gravity of the mother changes which affects not only posture but the stress on certain muscles that have to deal with the posture change.
	Diastasis recti	As a result of the abdomen swelling (due to the foetus) the tendon band that keeps the rectus abdominis muscle in place can split to allow for the growth. This is called diastasis recti.
	Ligament relaxation	Because of the increase in the hormone relaxin, the pubic symphysis (bones in the pubic region) can become less stable and cause pregnancy-related pelvic girdle pain (previously known as symphysis pubis dysfunction), and in some cases they can separate (known as diastasis symphysis pubis).

There are several glands that are located at various sites around the body. These glands secrete hormone messengers. The pineal and pituitary glands are located in the brain whereas the other glands and tissues are located at other sites around the body. All hormones have specific roles but can be thought of in simple terms as just messengers acting on specific tissues. The tissue on which a hormone messenger acts is known as a 'receptor site'.

Table 3.2 gives an overview of the common glands in the body and their function related to the release of hormone messengers that circu-late around the body to deliver certain informa-tion. Even though all of the hormones in the body play crucial individual roles, there are several main hormones that are affected during preg-nancy that the reader should be aware of. These include oestrogen, progesterone, prolactin, human chorionic gonadotropin (HCG), insulin, human placental lactogen and relaxin.

Oestrogen

This particular hormone is considered to be the primary female sex hormone (although it is present in men) and is released by the ovaries.

Table 3.2	Roles of common glands and tissues
Gland	**Function**
Pituitary	About the size of a pea and located at the base of the brain, this gland produces mainly trophic (meaning to feed) hormones for growth purposes and the maintenance of blood pressure, as well as prolactin for breast milk.
Pineal	This gland is also located in the brain and releases melatonin to help promote sleep patterns and seasonal functions.
Thyroid	One of the largest glands, the thyroid (Greek for 'shield' relating to the shape of the cartilage) is located in the neck and is mainly responsible for controlling metabolism (how quickly the body uses energy).
Parathyroid	There are normally four parathyroid glands located just behind the thyroid gland. These glands produce hormones that control bone growth by regulating calcium levels in the body (in the blood and bones).
Adrenal glands	The adrenal glands sit on top of the kidneys and produce adrenalin, cortisol and noradrenaline (mainly in response to stress) which are responsible for the increase in nutrient breakdown to provide energy.
Pancreas	The pancreas is an endocrine organ located in the digestive system. It is responsible for the release of insulin and glucagon into the bloodstream in order to help regulate blood sugar levels.
Testes and ovaries	These glands produce sex hormones such as testosterone, relaxin, progesterone and oestrogen to regulate reproductive function.

It is present in the body prior to pregnancy but increases by 20 to 30 times during pregnancy. It belongs to a group of hormones called steroid hormones which are only soluble in lipid (fat) for the purpose of transport in the body. These hormones take a reasonable amount of time to have an effect but that effect is usually long lasting. It is the main hormone related to the growth of the baby, the uterus – which increases about 20 times in size from the size of a fist to that of a very large watermelon – and the breasts. Oestrogen also promotes tissue growth in the body but may also encourage fluid retention leading to swelling (oedema). Breasts can increase up to twice their normal size and the heart, particularly the left ventricle, may increase by up to one-third in size under the influence of oestrogen.

Progesterone

As with oestrogen, progesterone is also classed as a steroid hormone. Progesterone is involved in the female menstrual cycle and belongs to a class of hormones known as 'progestogens'. One of the main advantages of this particular hormone is the resulting effect it has in relaxing smooth muscle (muscle that is not under voluntary control) within the body, in particular the smooth muscles in the blood vessel walls, which helps to cope with the increased blood volume that typically occurs during pregnancy. Without this muscular relaxing effect, blood pressure can easily become dangerously high for both mother-to-be and the foetus.

Unfortunately the disadvantage of progesterone is that it can also cause relaxation of the smooth muscle in the digestive tract, which can lead to an increased likelihood of constipation and haemorrhoids. It can also increase the body's

basal temperature (the temperature of the body at complete rest) for the first 20 weeks of pregnancy, which can be an issue especially if exercising as overheating of the mother and baby is a primary concern (see page 20).

Prolactin

Secreted by the pituitary gland and controlled by the hypothalamus, this hormone is a protein (peptide hormone) that is also known as 'luteo-tropic hormone' (LTH). Its main role is that it initiates milk production after birth of the baby when oestrogen and progesterone levels fall in the mother. In simple terms, it does this by stimulating the breasts to fill with milk after they have been suckled in preparation for the next feed. It is also thought that prolactin plays a role in helping to prevent further pregnancy while breastfeeding by suppressing the ovulatory cycle. However, breastfeeding is not a reliable form of contraception as evidenced by the not insignificant number of women who attend their 6-week postnatal check-up already pregnant again!

Human chorionic gonadotropin (HCG)

This is the only hormone in the body that is produced during pregnancy, first by the embryo and then later by the placenta. Detection of HCG in the urine is often used to identify pregnancy. HCG, along with low blood sugar levels, is largely responsible for the symptoms of nausea and sickness that are common in early pregnancy. HCG is also responsible for helping to maintain the function of the ovaries until the placenta takes over during the second trimester. It is also thought that HCG helps to stimulate the secretion of progesterone which enriches the uterus with a lining of blood vessels, sustaining the growing foetus.

Insulin

This particular hormone is produced by the pancreas (as well as other hormones such as glucagon) and is a type of water-soluble hormone which is known as a peptide hormone. As a response to high blood sugar levels, insulin is normally secreted into the bloodstream which has the effect of reducing the blood sugar back to a normal level. This occurs during normal circumstances but in some cases does not work effectively during pregnancy (in some cases it can reduce blood sugar to dangerously low levels).

Pregnant women can also display high blood sugar levels, especially during the third trimester, but insulin resistance can also increase (meaning blood sugar levels will stay high) during pregnancy which makes a pregnant woman's energy utilisation similar to that of a mild diabetic (see page 24 for more information on gestational diabetes).

Human placental lactogen

This hormone is similar (in structure and function) to human growth hormone. It is produced by the placenta and is essential for foetal development as it helps to regulate energy supply. It is also used for preparation/stimulation of milk production.

Relaxin

Known as a protein hormone, relaxin is produced initially by the ovaries up to about 12–14 weeks, and then by the placenta during pregnancy. Although this particular hormone is still under investigation it is thought that relaxin affects the collagen fibres of all connective tissue in the body. For example, it makes connective tissue in ligaments and tendons more pliable and elastic, making joints less stable. This includes relaxing the connective tissue that supports the sacroiliac joint and pubic symphysis which destabilises the pelvic girdle, however, the advantage of this is that it allows the pelvic outlet to widen ready for delivery. All other joints in the body are also affected and therefore range of movement is increased.

It has been shown that relaxin levels in the mother-to-be appear to peak at about week 14 into the pregnancy and then again around delivery time. Production of relaxin then tends to cease once the baby is delivered, but the effects of the hormone can remain for some time afterwards. Joints therefore can remain slightly unstable for about five months postnatally and if the mother is also breast-feeding then it can be even longer as levels dissipate more slowly when feeding. It is also generally understood that levels of relaxin will be increased in the second or subsequent pregnancies, leading to increased effects of joint instability. There are also other effects which are thought to include the following:

- Reduction of blood clotting: Women may bruise more easily or bleed more profusely from a wound.
- Reduction of uterine activity: The uterus contracts throughout the normal menstrual cycle and this reduces when pregnant to help maintain the pregnancy.
- Inhibition of histamine release: This may reduce symptoms or occurrence of hay fever during pregnancy.
- Preparation of cervix for labour: Allows the cervix to 'ripen' and dilate fully to allow the baby to be born.

In terms of the effect of hormones released during pregnancy in relation to exercise, there are many precautions that should be taken, but it is the

Table 3.3	Mechanisms of heat loss and gain
Mechanism of heat loss	**Mechanism of heat gain**
Metabolic heat (chemical reactions in the body)	Radiation
Conduction and convection	Conduction and convection
Radiation	Evaporation

effect of relaxin on the ligaments that is most crucial. This needs to be taken into account with any exercise programme. It is therefore important for instructors to have an understanding of the properties and functions of ligaments and the main ones that contribute to the stability of joints in the body.

THERMOREGULATION CHANGES

Even though variations in environmental temperature can affect body temperature, there are various internal mechanisms that can also have an effect. This is especially so during pregnancy as hormonal influence can increase body temperature (see page 12). It is important for instructors to understand how the body regulates temperature, a process known as 'thermoregulation'.

When discussing thermoregulation the term 'homeostasis' (*homoios* meaning 'the same' and *stasis* meaning 'still') is often closely associated. Homeostasis is described as 'the condition in which the body's internal environment remains within certain physiological limits' (Tortora and Grabowski, 1996, *Principles of Anatomy and Physiology*). In relation to pregnancy and exercise this simply means that the systems within the body try to maintain the temperature within limits as they do in any other situation.

Human beings can be classified as being 'homeothermic' (*homoios* meaning 'the same' and

Heat Loss + Gain: Terminology
- Conduction: Transfer of heat between two bodies (solid, liquid or gas) that are in direct contact. Heat flows down the thermal gradient.
- Convection: Heat transfer by the movement of a fluid (liquid or gas). Depends on movement of liquids.
- Radiation: Heat transfer between two bodies not in direct contact.
- Evaporation: Vaporisation of fluid at the skin's surface.
- Metabolic heat: Heat generated by the body's internal chemical activity.

therm meaning 'heat'), which simply means that the body's systems continually work to keep the internal temperature between 36.1 and 37.8°C. This is not always possible as body temperature can change under extreme conditions such as heavy exercise, illness, extreme heat or cold.

In practical terms, during exercise the body will heat up. It needs to lose this heat otherwise hyperthermia (excessively high body temperature) can occur. In normal situations the body is relatively good at balancing heat losses with heat production in order to prevent hyperthermia or hypothermia (excessively low body temperature). The body can either gain heat energy (get warmer) or lose heat energy (get colder) as a result of various internal and external mechanisms. Although there are many complex factors associated with heat gain and heat loss within the human body, table 3.3 shows the main contributing factors that can affect the thermoregulation of an individual.

Heat gain

Any form of physical activity or exercise that a person is taking part in, depending on the intensity at which it is performed, can have the effect of increasing the metabolic rate (this can be described as the amount of energy expended at a particular time) by as much as 15–20 times that of normal resting rate, which is known as the 'basal metabolic rate' (BMR). Also, the increased muscle contraction that occurs during exercise creates a large amount of heat because when muscles contract, 70–75 per cent of the energy that is produced is released as heat. The body needs to find some way to lose this excess heat because if it didn't, core temperature in the body would reach fatal levels within a matter of a few minutes. As one of the effects of increased progesterone levels during pregnancy is to raise the core body temperature, it is important to ensure that intensity is at an appropriate level to avoid overheating, or hyperthermia, as thermoregulation may be compromised.

Heat loss

When the body gains heat as a result of exercise there needs to be some kind of heat loss in order to compensate. This can occur by various means such as convection, radiation, conduction

Table 3.4	Mechanisms of heat loss at rest and during exercise	
Mechanism	% loss at rest	% loss exercising
Conduction and convection	20	15
Radiation	60	5
Evaporation	20	80+

or evaporation (as shown in table 3.4). However, the amount that each of these contributes to heat loss varies depending on several factors. For instance, environmental conditions (both hot and cold weather), the intensity of the exercise and the clothing worn by the individual can all influence how heat is lost.

Conduction and convection normally account for about 10–20 per cent of heat loss at rest and slightly less during exercise. Radiation from the body however (through infrared rays) accounts for about 60 per cent of heat loss at rest but drops to minimal levels during exercise. The main mechanism of heat loss during exercise is through fluid evaporation, mainly in the form of sweating, which accounts for up to 80–90 per cent of total heat loss.

Although all the various mechanisms of heat loss contribute to some degree at rest and during exercise, the percentages of contribution differ greatly. It can be seen in table 3.4 that at rest, radiation is the main mechanism of heat loss whereas during exercise, evaporation of sweat becomes the main mechanism.

In simple terms, during exercise heat loss is mainly achieved by a process known as vasodilation (widening of blood vessels supplying the skin). This widening causes an increase in blood flow to the surface of the body which then leads to the familiar reddening of the skin and sweating.

It should also be remembered that the greater the difference in temperature between the skin (~34°C) and the environment that the individual is in, the greater is the amount of heat lost through radiation. For example, heat loss is much greater if an individual is exercising in a cold environment than in a warm environment because the temperature difference between the individual and the environment is greater. If the exercise becomes more intense then evaporation becomes the major contributor to heat loss as a result of an increase in sweating.

All of the systems in the body that help to regulate body temperature are controlled by the hypothalamus (Greek meaning 'under' and 'chamber', as it sits under the thalamus within the brain). As well as thermoregulation, the hypothalamus is responsible for controlling other functions in the body such as hunger, thirst and sleep. The hypothalamus receives information regarding body temperature and responds to this by either conserving or dissipating body heat. If the temperature of the body increases (too hot) the following responses take place in order to help prevent a further rise in temperature (and to initiate cooling processes) as shown in figure 3.2.

Did you know?

Being a heavy sweater can be a sign of fitness. Fitter individuals can exercise at higher intensities, resulting in more heat production, and will start sweating earlier and with a greater amount than unfit people. Also, it is quite common for people to sweat as much as 1–2.5L/h (litres per hour). Even though evaporation of 1L of sweat can dissipate a large amount of heat (580kcal), with heavy sweating or in humid conditions some of the sweat produced often drops off the body without evaporating, thus removing much of the benefit in terms of thermoregulation. There are approximately 3–4 million sweat glands that can be found on the skin of a human body. Sweat is mainly made up of water with a small amount of electrolytes (any substance containing free ions) dissolved within it. The volume of sweat produced by an individual can be affected by several factors such as exercise intensity, environmental conditions, fitness, hydration levels and heat acclimatisation.

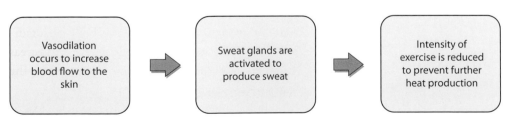

Figure 3.2 Cooling processes within the body

Exercise in warm environments

It is important that pregnant women are aware of the effects of exercise in hot and humid conditions because of the potential dangers of overheating. In normal exercise situations during pregnancy, the circulatory system (the heart and associated vessels) is responsible for the regulation of the transfer of heat from working muscles (caused by the repetitive contraction and relaxation of muscles which is known as the hysteresis effect) to the surface of the body, via the dilated blood vessels, for heat loss purposes. As a result, the amount of blood pumped out of the heart with each beat (stroke volume) and the heart rate increase in order to do this. This reduces the oxygen flow to the foetus which can have severe effects if it is prolonged. When exercising in warm or humid conditions, thermoregulation can be less effective resulting in a more rapid overheating which can obviously become dangerous if not dealt with. In these particular conditions the rate of sweating can increase due to the saturated nature of the surrounding air, which can prevent the evaporation of sweat from the surface of the body. If an individual in this situation continues to exercise, the risk of heat injury increases rapidly due to dehydration and the inability of the body to cool down. Heat injury can lead to symptoms such as cramps, exhaustion and in severe cases heat stroke and even death.

CARDIOVASCULAR CHANGES

The familiar term 'cardiovascular' simply means to do with the heart and the vessels that are associated with it. Many changes occur within this system from conception, during pregnancy and for some time afterwards. For example, as there is a demand for increased oxygen levels to supply the foetus as well as the mother-to-be, the body responds by increasing the amount of blood in the system (known as blood volume) in order to carry more oxygen. It has been shown that during pregnancy this can increase by as much as 50 per cent more than normal levels (Guyton and Hall, 2005).

However, even though the amount of blood in the body increases, because more oxygen is needed, the body produces more red blood cells, which are the cells that transport the oxygen in the blood (oxygen is actually attached to a part of the cell known as 'haemoglobin'). The number of red blood cells can increase by as much as 20–30 per cent in order to supply the increased oxygen to the foetus and mother-to-be.

Although red blood cells increase during pregnancy, the greater increase in plasma volume can in some cases lead to a type of anaemia called 'physiological anaemia'. In the non-pregnant state, a reduction of iron in the body results in smaller, paler red blood cells being produced, causing a reduction in their oxygen-carrying capacity. If iron stores are used and not replenished then anaemia can occur.

During pregnancy, however, the cause of anaemia is slightly different. Both the mother-

Did you know?

The greatest incidence of heat exhaustion in the Great North Run, the world's biggest half-marathon held in Newcastle in the UK, was when a celebrity fitness instructor encouraged many of the 50,000 entrants to perform a vigorous warm-up on what was already a warm day.

Table 3.5	Typical blood volume levels in both non-pregnant and pregnant women	
Blood component	**Non-pregnant**	**Pregnant, full term**
Total blood volume	4000ml	5500ml
Plasma volume	2600ml	3850ml
Red blood cell mass	1400ml	1650ml
Haemoglobin	12.5–13.9g/dL	11.0–12.2g/dL

Adapted from Medforth et al (2006)

to-be and the foetus need iron, however there is a relative reduction in the concentration of iron and red blood cells in the bloodstream due to an increased dilation of blood vessels, brought about by progesterone combined with the increase in blood plasma needed to maintain a healthy blood pressure. As plasma increases, so too do the levels of red and white blood cells (these help to fight infection) and platelets (these help the blood to clot). As the increased amount of plasma becomes greater than that of the cells, a condition known as 'haemodilution' occurs, which is one of the conditions that can lead to physiological anaemia. There is however an advantage to haemodilution as there is a beneficial response in that it helps the perfusion (or delivery of blood and nutrients) of blood flow through the placenta, which is considered relatively normal in pregnancy. Although the World Health Organization (WHO) recommends that haemoglobin levels should remain above 11.0g/dL (grams per decilitre), levels below this are often considered by some to require iron supplementation. Table 3.5 gives an overview of typical blood volume levels in both non-pregnant and pregnant women.

As a result of the increase in the amount of blood in the body, the size of the blood vessels increases to allow this greater volume of blood to be able to flow around the body. This increase in blood vessel diameter is stimulated by the hormone progesterone (see page 15) and is known as 'vasodilation'. However a disadvantage of this is that it can lead to a fall in blood pressure below normal levels, which means that blood might not be pumped around the body as well as it should. This is known as 'vascular underfill' and it has been shown that regular exercise can help to minimise this effect.

Vascular underfill

As progesterone causes relaxation and increased elasticity of blood vessel walls there may be a short period in early pregnancy prior to the increase in blood volume where there is in effect a reduced volume of blood circulating, which makes it hard to maintain optimum blood pressure. This is known as 'vascular underfill' and may lead to dizziness and light-headedness when standing for longer than a few minutes or when changing from a lying to seated or seated to standing position. Known as postural or 'orthostatic hypotension', this means that care should be taken to avoid sudden changes in position or standing still for more than a minute or two in the first trimester.

Early on in the pregnancy, resting heart rate increases by as much as 10–15bpm. It does this in order to deliver the increased demand for oxygen, which means that the amount of blood pumped out of the heart every minute can increase by as much as 30 per cent. This amount of blood pumped out every minute is known as the 'cardiac output'.

Note: It was mentioned earlier that the amount of blood pumped out of the heart every beat is called the 'stroke volume'. Because cardiac output is the amount pumped out of the heart every minute and heart rate is the number of beats every minute, it follows that:

> Cardiac output = stroke volume x heart rate (measured in litres per minute)

One of the reasons that the heart is able to pump more blood out with each beat is that the size of the heart chamber that pumps the blood around the body (known as the left ventricle) can enlarge by about 20 per cent to help cope with the increased demand placed upon it. Exercise can also help in that it can make the heart stronger, since it is a muscle (it is actually 'cardiac' muscle). The larger chamber and the stronger cardiac muscle in combination results in a greater amount of blood being pumped every beat.

There are also changes that occur during pregnancy, however, that are known to have associated risks. For example, the liver increases the production of certain chemicals, such as fibrinogen and factor VIII (FVIII), which cause the blood to clot more easily (known as hypercoagulability). This, along with a more sedentary lifestyle before and during the term of a pregnancy, can increase the risk of blood clots and deep vein thrombosis

(DVT) for the mother-to-be. It has also been suggested that women are at their highest risk for developing clots, or thrombi, during the weeks following the birth (postnatal period). Clots more commonly occur in the left leg where the left iliac vein is crossed by the right iliac artery. This occurs as the increased blood flow in the right iliac artery of the mother after birth compresses the left iliac vein leading to an increased risk of thrombosis (clotting), which is often made worse by the lack of mobility following delivery. For these reasons, it is recommended that all women actively engage in regular exercise prior to, throughout the duration, and resume appropriate activity as soon as possible after a pregnancy in order to minimise the potential for clotting.

RESPIRATORY CHANGES

The term 'respiratory', for the purpose of this book, relates to the lungs and the associated vessels. During pregnancy there are many changes within the cardiovascular system which result in an increased demand to deliver more oxygen via the blood, which is why the respiratory system has to adapt in order to help to cope with this. Another reason why respiratory changes are needed is that total lung capacity can be reduced by the pressure of the enlarged uterus on the diaphragm of the mother-to-be.

One of the first changes to occur during pregnancy is that the brain (of the mother-to-be) becomes more sensitive to carbon dioxide which has the effect of increasing the breathing rate (the hormone progesterone is responsible for this). Care must be taken, as an increased breathing rate can lead to hyperventilation (sometimes known as 'over breathing') which is common at about 12 weeks into the pregnancy.

Did you know?

Hyperventilation can constrict blood vessels to the brain. It does this when more carbon dioxide is breathed out than is produced in the body. This changes the acidity (pH) in the blood, which then causes constriction. The body tries to compensate for this rise in blood pH by increased excretion of bicarbonate via the urine, to maintain a normal pH balance.

One advantage of the increase in breathing rate is that the amount of air taken in and out of the lungs (this is known as 'tidal volume') increases by about 40–50 per cent.

All individuals have a type of 'reserve' space in the lungs which is known as the 'residual volume'. This is essentially the capacity or volume in the lungs that is not normally used. During pregnancy, this residual volume normally becomes less, therefore there is more lung capacity than can be used. The increase in the breathing rate combined with the increase in the available capacity means that more oxygen can be delivered to the blood vessels. However, when we breathe in, not all of the oxygen in the air is used up, but during pregnancy this amount can increase by as much as 30 per cent.

METABOLIC CHANGES

For the purpose of this book, the term 'metabolism' will simply refer to all the chemical reactions that take place in the body at a cellular level. For instance, basal metabolic rate (BMR) as mentioned previously can be simply defined as 'the amount of energy used by all the chemical reactions in the body at rest' (this is normally measured in kilocalories or kcals). The amount of energy used by the body at rest (BMR) has been shown to increase by as much as 20 per cent during pregnancy (for obvious reasons discussed throughout this book).

In terms of the type of fuel that is used (a better term is 'metabolised') in the body to provide energy, there is often a high usage of carbohydrate (often referred to as sugar when it is digested) by the foetus, which means that the mother-to-be should be encouraged to eat carbohydrate-based snacks on a regular basis to avoid 'sugar' lows (when carbohydrate is broken down it releases sugar in forms such as glucose, fructose and galactose). If the mother-to-be does not snack regularly, sugar lows would typically occur about every 6–8 hours due to the usage by the foetus.

It has been commonly demonstrated that carbohydrate metabolism is affected by the foetal/placental unit in many ways including the following:

- Fall in fasting blood glucose from week 10
- Human placental lactogen increases maternal resistance to insulin
- Post-meal blood glucose levels are higher and remain higher after meals
- Resulting increase in insulin requirement triggers a three- to four-fold increase in insulin release
- Pancreatic cells become overworked
- Fat stores are used, which raises free fatty acid and glycerol levels and induces ketosis (a build-up of ketones in the blood which raise acidity levels).

To compound this problem, pregnant women also display a delayed insulin response which can lead to a mild form of diabetes throughout the pregnancy (see page 24). Remember: Insulin is the hormone that is released by the pancreas (an organ in the stomach area) which reduces the amount of sugar in the bloodstream if it goes too high. If this system does not work effectively, it means blood sugar can become too high (a condition known as 'hyperglycaemia') and put excessive strain on the heart. If this persists it can result in a condition known as 'gestational diabetes' (GD), which is a form of glucose intolerance that occurs during pregnancy and which usually resolves after birth. Figures generally state that between 3 and 12 per cent of pregnant women will develop GD, but it is important to understand that the condition can cause an increased risk of future diabetes to mother and baby. For example, the American College of Sports Medicine (ACSM) have stated that approximately 50 per cent of the women who develop GD develop Type 2 diabetes later in life even though the reasons are not fully understood.

GD is normally diagnosed using an oral glucose tolerance test, usually done after an overnight fast. This process involves ingesting a glucose drink containing a standard amount of glucose (75g). Blood samples are taken before the drink is given and two hours later. Specific blood glucose levels are then used to identify GD. Women who have been diagnosed with GD will need to be monitored during the pregnancy and may experience more frequent hypoglycaemic episodes. This is another reason to encourage regular carbohydrate snacks such as fresh fruit and vegetables rather than processed sugar-type snacks such as cakes and biscuits.

Weight gain

One of the other main metabolic changes during pregnancy is that of weight gain as discussed previously. The increase in the hormone oestrogen throughout pregnancy has been shown to increase the resting metabolic rate of the mother-to-be by as much as 20 per cent. This is often misinterpreted as permission to 'eat for two' but in reality this only allows for about an extra 300kcal per day (and that should only be after the first trimester). Any additional calorie intake beyond this will typically be stored as maternal fat and may prove hard to lose after the birth.

Guidelines typically state that the emphasis in the first trimester is on a healthy, balanced diet, nausea and sickness permitting, with a recommended first trimester weight gain of approximately 1–3kg, or 10 per cent of the total pregnancy weight gain. The greatest weight gain usually occurs in the second trimester when an average gain of 6–8kg is recommended. By the third trimester, weight gain is relatively slow and steady at approximately 3.5–4kg. Weight gain of less than 1kg per month in the third trimester

Table 3.6	Recommended weight gain by body mass index (BMI)	
Pre-pregnancy BMI	Recommended weight gain	
	kg	lbs
Low < 19.8	12.5–18	28–40
Normal 19.8–26	11.5–16	25–35
Overweight 26–29	7–11.5	15–25
Obese > 30	5–9	11–20

Adapted from Medforth et al (2006)

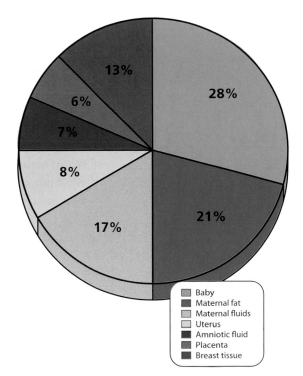

Legend:
- Baby
- Maternal fat
- Maternal fluids
- Uterus
- Amniotic fluid
- Placenta
- Breast tissue

Figure 3.3 Optimal weight gain in pregnancy based on 12kg/26lbs total gain (adapted from Wolfe (2005))

GASTROINTESTINAL CHANGES

One of the more common symptoms of pregnancy (this particular symptom affects more than half of all pregnant women) is nausea and vomiting, which is more commonly referred to as 'morning sickness' but the correct term that should be used is 'nausea gravidarum'. Women typically start to experience this around week 6 and it often disappears by about week 12.

The effects of nausea can be quite mild but they can also be quite severe. If this is the case then vomiting may lead to dehydration and subsequent weight loss. It tends to be present in the early hours of the morning and reduces as the day progresses. Some women, however, find that the symptoms come on at different times of day and in some cases can even be present all of the time!

It is generally thought that the nauseous symptoms may be linked to increased levels of oestrogen and HCG and possibly low blood sugar levels, although research continues to be done in this area. Another possible suggestion that has been put forward is that morning sickness is linked to a safety response from the mother-to-be. For example, there is evidence by Flaxman and Sherman (2000) that suggests that morning sick-

may be a cause for clinical concern and should be reported to clinical staff as soon as possible. The emphasis is still on a healthy, balanced diet with an extra (quality) 300kcal per day.

Table 3.6 gives a brief overview of the recommended weight gain as classified by pre-pregnancy body mass index (see appendix 4 on page 174 for an explanation of body mass index).

It is interesting to know that during pregnancy the associated weight gain is distributed between several places. The largest gain tends to be the mother's fat tissue and of course the baby itself. Figure 3.3 shows what is considered to be the ideal weight gain distribution based on a healthy weight gain of 12kg.

Did you know?

Thalidomide was a sedative drug developed in Germany in the 1950s and was prescribed as a cure for morning sickness in many countries. It was withdrawn from the market in 1961 when the drug's effects came to light (it caused birth defects such as affecting the growth of limbs in foetuses).

25

ness is often triggered by animal products including meat and fish which contain parasites and harmful bacteria that would be especially dangerous to pregnant women. Whatever the cause, symptoms of nausea and vomiting can be inconvenient at best and hugely troublesome at worst.

Another gastrointestinal effect brought on by increased levels of progesterone during pregnancy is that of the relaxation of smooth muscle such as the 'gastroesophageal sphincter', which can lead to acid reflux, a condition where stomach acid comes up into the throat (Note: smooth muscle is a type of muscle in the body that is controlled by the autonomic nervous system; in other words it contracts without conscious control). The relaxation of smooth muscle tissue within the digestive system can also lead to constipation as the system becomes more sluggish. Another of the effects is that stools can become dried out and harder, making them difficult or painful to pass. If this is the case it can in turn lead to rectal haemorrhoids (piles) which may start to form early in pregnancy and can remain long after the baby has been delivered.

A further effect of increased levels of progesterone on the GI system is the onset, or increased levels of heartburn and/or indigestion. This condition can occur particularly in the first trimester although nausea is more likely at this time. The combination of heartburn or indigestion and nausea or sickness can lead to disrupted eating patterns for the mother-to-be, which can result in low energy levels or even weight loss in the first trimester.

POSTURAL AND MUSCULOSKELETAL CHANGES

The main change in relation to posture comes as a result of the body having to adapt to the change in the centre of gravity. Generally speaking, the centre of gravity in a person lies at the level of the naval just in front of the spine, however, as a baby gets bigger during pregnancy, it causes the centre of gravity of the mother-to-be to move. In the case of a pregnant woman, the baby is growing outwards therefore this causes the centre of gravity to move outwards and also slightly down. As a result of this shift in the centre of gravity, there are several negative postural effects that can occur which can eventually lead to back pain in many cases. These postural effects include:

- the lengthening and weakening of abdominal muscles;
- ligaments loosening mainly around the hips, lower back and pelvis;
- reduced support for the spine as a result of weakened muscles;
- an increased lumbar lordosis (hollow lower back) and an increased thoracic kyphosis (rounded upper back) as an additional result of this weakness and
- a further increase in the lumbar curve due to the pelvis being tilted forward.

The pregnant woman typically displays a different pattern of gait (the term for a walking or running pattern). The step or stride lengthens as the pregnancy progresses, as a result of the weight gain and changes in posture. It is interesting to note that on average, a woman's foot can grow by a half size or more during pregnancy. In addition, the combined effect of an increase in body weight during pregnancy, fluid retention and weight gain lowers the arches of the foot, further adding to the foot's length and

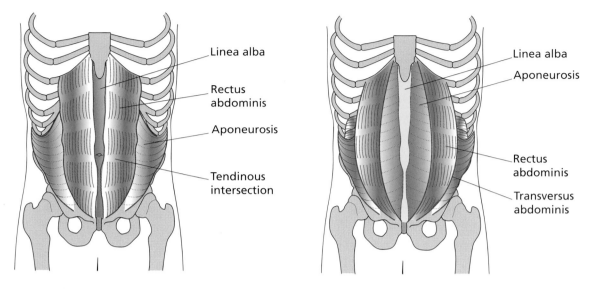

Figure 3.4 Abdominal wall before and after diastasis recti

width. In later stages of pregnancy this may result in the typical 'waddling' gait seen in many pregnant women.

Diastasis recti

One of the main abdominal muscles that is often affected by pregnancy is the rectus abdominis (often referred to as the 'six-pack'), which runs from both sides of the lower ribs in a vertical line down to the pelvic bone. During pregnancy this muscle lengthens and also becomes wider. When this occurs the muscle might appear to split down the middle as can be seen in figure 3.4 but it is actually a band of tendon (or aponeurosis) called the 'linea alba' which separates to allow for growth of the baby and swelling of the abdomen area. This separation of the rectus abdominis muscle is otherwise known as 'diastasis recti' and occurs in about two-thirds of all pregnant women.

Pelvic girdle pain

During pregnancy the sacroiliac joint (between the sacrum and the ilium) and the sacrococcygeal joint (between the sacrum and the coccyx) become loose to allow the symphysis pubis to widen for the prospective birth (an increase of 3–4mm is considered to be normal). However, in the later stages of pregnancy this widening can increase to as much as 9mm or more which compromises the stability of the pelvic girdle (and can also affect pelvic stability after delivery) and can lead to pain in the lower back, the pubic area and down into the legs where it may be mistaken for sciatica. This specific pain is referred to as 'pregnancy-related pelvic girdle pain' (PGP) and while this is a relatively common occurrence in pregnancy (experienced by up to 45 per cent of pregnant women) it is not considered to be 'normal'. PGP can cause pain at the front or back of the pelvis and lead to problems with walking, everyday activities and weight-bearing on one leg such as when walking upstairs or getting in and out of cars or bed. Almost any movement of the hips can cause discomfort or pain so it is important to try and minimise this discomfort by keeping the hips aligned and stable. Taking shorter walking strides, avoiding crossing the legs or adduction at the hip, keeping activity low impact and short duration are all strategies that can help to minimise the pain.

There are no easily identifiable risk factors for PGP, however a previous history of injury or trauma to the pelvis, low back pain or PGP may increase the risk. Other potential risk factors include second or subsequent pregnancies, heavy physical work or activity, obesity or joint hyper mobility so it is important to screen for these prior to commencing an exercise programme with a pregnant client. An extreme separation of 10mm to 35mm, known as 'diastasis symphysis pubis' (DSP) needs careful consideration as it can lead to long-term problems with pelvic girdle stability. Diagnosed by clinical investigation, DSP may cause considerable discomfort or pain and any exercise will need to ensure the pelvis is correctly aligned to avoid exacerbating this.

Risk factors for DSP include prior pelvic trauma, PGP and traumatic or quick birth, particularly if the baby has a large head circumference.

The pelvic floor

The so called 'pelvic floor' is a complex structure of muscles and connective tissue that plays an important role in continence, sexual function and in supporting the pelvic and abdominal organs, particularly the uterus during pregnancy. The pelvic floor consists of two groups or layers of muscles: the levator ani and the coccygeus (see figure 3.5).

The levator ani, which constitutes the largest and deepest layer of the pelvic floor, consists of the pubococcygeus, puborectalis and iliococcygeus

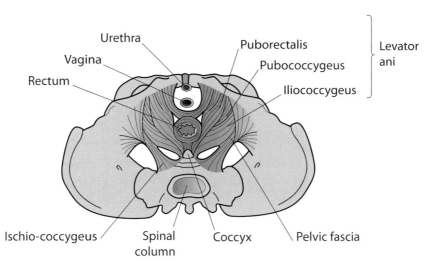

Figure 3.5 Muscles of the pelvic floor

muscles. As a group, these muscles act together to lift and tighten the pelvic floor. The coccygeus is the superficial (closest to the surface) layer and lies at the back of the levator ani. Most of the pelvic floor muscle fibres, around 70 per cent, are slow-twitch to provide continuous support (an endurance role) for the organs, while the remaining 30 per cent or so have a fast-twitch function, contracting rapidly in response to sudden increases in intra-abdominal pressure. Pelvic floor exercises are particularly important during pregnancy as the weight of the growing uterus and the effects of the hormone relaxin can weaken these muscles and lead to acute and chronic stress incontinence both while pregnant and following delivery.

It is estimated that over two-thirds of women experience stress incontinence during pregnancy and it is still present in up to 38 per cent two to three months after delivery. It is also estimated that up to one in three of all women (who are not pregnant) over the age of 40 suffer with stress incontinence and just 'put up with it' yet research shows that regular performance of pelvic floor exercises may be effective in reducing this particular condition (Mørkved 2007). A strong and healthy pelvic floor is also capable of stretching more easily than a weak one during delivery and will also return to normal more quickly after delivery, particularly if exercises are performed in the immediate postnatal period. Part 3 gives guidelines for exercising this particular muscle group.

Common ligaments in the body

As mentioned throughout this book, during pregnancy there is an increased release of a hormone called relaxin. The effect of this particular hormone is thought (research in this area is still uncertain) to loosen ligaments throughout the pregnancy and up to six months postnatally. Even though it is still under debate as to whether this actually occurs or not, it is advisable to err on the side of caution. Because of the shift in centre of gravity and the possible effect of the relaxin, the loose ligaments supporting the pelvis, hips and lower back can stretch leading to decreased stability and increased stress on the joints. It is important therefore that muscles around the trunk and hips are kept as strong as possible and that any flexibility exercises at this point are stopped or done with extreme caution.

In terms of their structure, ligaments are found throughout the body and are tough, white, fibrous (mainly collagen) tissues with a poor blood supply that are strung together in a strap-like formation. They are generally attached from bone to bone and their function is to allow wanted movement while preventing unwanted movement around joints. Ligaments have only a very slight elastic property and if damaged in any way, the healing time of the ligament is quite slow (usually several weeks) due to the poor blood supply available. In addition, depending on the severity or grade of the damage to the ligament, it can take several months for the healing process to complete. Ligaments can however become stronger and in some cases hypertrophy (become larger) following weight-bearing activities that are essential for joint stability.

Ligaments of the abdomen

The uterus is held in place in the abdomen by ligaments, including those known as 'round ligaments'. During pregnancy, as the uterus increases in both size and weight, the round ligaments are placed under increasing stress as they lengthen and this can pull on nerves and tissues causing a type of pain known as 'round ligament pain'. This pain can vary from mild to severe and may cause worry despite being a relatively normal occurrence in pregnancy. Round ligament pain can be caused by sudden movements such as changing position in bed, by exercise or can just be due to the growth of the uterus. While round ligament pain is a relatively normal experience in pregnancy, any severe or prolonged pain in the abdomen should always be checked out by a medical professional so if the mother-to-be mentions unusual or increased pains, recommend she discusses this with her antenatal care provider.

Ligaments of the pelvis

The pelvis is a key structure in pregnancy and the effects of relaxin on the ligaments of the sacroiliac joint and the symphysis pubis can cause widening of the pelvic outlet and separation of the symphysis pubis. There are no muscle attachments across the sacroiliac or pubic joints and so they are dependent on ligaments for stability. Cartilage lines the surfaces of the joints and a pad of cartilage between the pubic bones, at the symphysis pubis, acts as support, shock absorption and to maintain stability and alignment of the pelvis.

Ligaments of the hip

The main functions of the hip joint are flexion, extension, abduction, adduction and a certain amount of rotation (see appendix 1 on page 170 for an explanation of all movements). The ligaments found in the hip joint are the:

* Iliofemoral ligament
* Pubofemoral ligament
* Ischiofemoral ligament

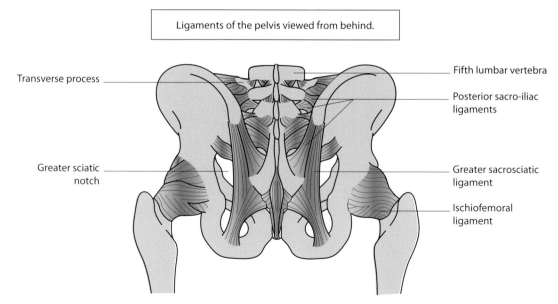

Ligaments of the pelvis viewed from behind.

Transverse process

Greater sciatic notch

Fifth lumbar vertebra

Posterior sacro-iliac ligaments

Greater sacrosciatic ligament

Ischiofemoral ligament

Figure 3.6 Common ligaments of the pelvis

As the hip joint is classed as a freely moveable synovial joint, it requires a certain degree of movement in all directions. The ligament structures in the hip joint allow this degree of movement but also provide a certain amount of stability at the end ranges and prevent the femur from pulling out of its socket, the acetabulum (this is known as a 'luxation'). During pregnancy these ligaments allow the hip joint to be more flexible so that the legs can open wider for childbirth. Therefore it is essential that strengthening of the hip joint muscles takes place in order to provide a degree of stability.

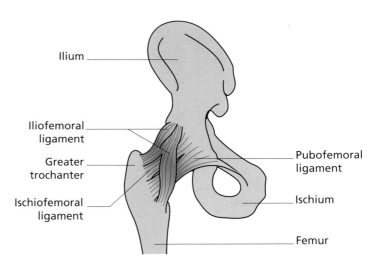

Figure 3.7 Common ligaments of the hip

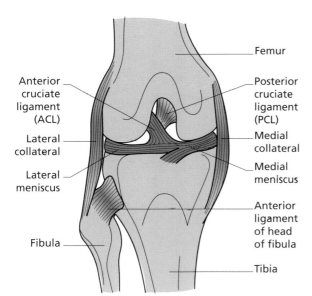

Figure 3.8 Common ligaments of the knee

Ligaments of the knee

The main function of the knee is flexion and extension with a slight degree of rotation. The ligaments found in the knee joint are the:

- Medial collateral ligament
- Lateral collateral ligament
- Anterior cruciate ligament
- Posterior cruciate ligament

The medial and lateral collateral ligaments are located on the medial (inside) and lateral (outside) aspects of the knee joint for the purpose of allowing knee flexion and extension and preventing any other movement. The anterior (front) and posterior (back) cruciate ligaments are located within the knee joint between the femur and tibia to prevent the two bones from sliding away from each other.

Ligaments of the shoulder

The main ligaments found in the shoulder joint (glenohumeral) are the:

* Coracohumeral ligament
* Glenohumeral (superior, middle and inferior) ligaments
* Coracoacromial ligament

As the shoulder joint is classed a freely moveable synovial joint, it requires a certain degree of movement in all directions (flexion, extension, abduction, adduction, rotation and circumduction). The ligament structures in the shoulder joint allow this wide range of movement but provide stability at the end ranges and prevent the humerus from pulling out of its socket, the glenoid cavity (another example of a luxation).

Ligaments of the ankle

Ligaments of the ankle can be separated into medial and lateral groups. The names of the ligaments are taken from the bones to which they attach so that they can easily be identified. The medial ligaments are a group of ligaments called the deltoids which are comprised of the following:

* Calcaneotibial (between calcaneous and tibia)
* Anterior and posterior talotibial (between talus and tibia)
* Tibionavicular (between tibia and navicular)

The lateral ligaments known as the lateral collateral ligaments are made up of the following:

* Calcaneofibular (between the calcaneus and the fibula)

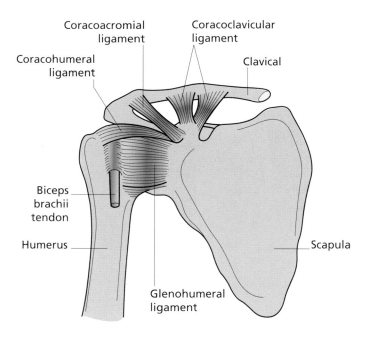

Figure 3.9 Common ligaments of the shoulder

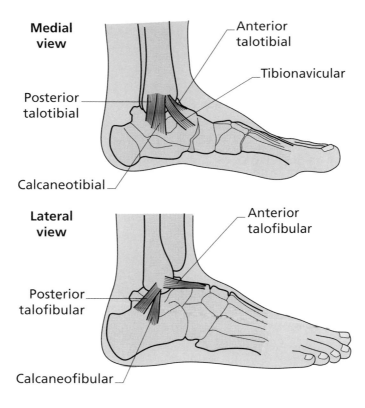

Medial view

Anterior talotibial

Tibionavicular

Posterior talotibial

Calcaneotibial

Lateral view

Anterior talofibular

Posterior talofibular

Calcaneofibular

Figure 3.10 Common ligaments of the ankle

• Anterior and posterior talofibular (between the talus and the fibula)

The deltoid and lateral collateral ligaments between them allow the foot to move quite freely in flexion and extension but provide the main stability in lateral movements such as inversion and eversion (see appendix 1, page 170). In other words, they prevent the ankle from rolling in or out which would easily lead to injury.

During pregnancy relaxin affects the ligaments in the ankle causing the feet to spread and it is not uncommon for a woman to go up one, or even more, shoe sizes.

OTHER EFFECTS AS A RESULT OF CHANGES DURING PREGNANCY

As well as the common changes that occur, there are a number of other symptoms that the instructor should be aware of.

Carpal tunnel syndrome (CTS)

This condition (not exclusive to pregnancy) is caused by the pressure of oedema (fluid retention) on the medial nerve in the wrist and can lead to numbness, tingling or pain in the wrist, thumbs, index and middle fingers. It is most commonly experienced during the night and may affect grip strength or be caused by excessive wrist positions, therefore caution must be taken when using resistance machines or hand-held free weights. It appears to be more common after delivery but does occur during the pregnancy.

Leg cramps
It is estimated that about one-third of women experience leg cramps during pregnancy so stretching during, as well as before and after, exercise may help to alleviate this.

Chloasma
Sometimes referred to as the 'mask of pregnancy', this particular condition can cause darker pigmentation on the face and especially around the eyes. If exercising outside, recommend your client to use a sunscreen or wear a hat to prevent this worsening. Chloasma does not appear to have any effect on exercise other than causing embarrassment to the mother-to-be in public situations if it is pronounced.

Stretch marks
The increased level of hormones during pregnancy combined with the growth of the uterus may lead to stretch marks which can be upsetting for the mother-to-be, particularly if they are severe.

Hair
For many women, pregnancy can lead to either a reduction in hair loss or an increase in hair growth, which leads to a head of full and healthy hair. However, increased hair growth can also occur on the face and arms, which may cause distress, particularly if it is excessive or perceived as unsightly.

Hyperemesis gravidarum (HG)
This condition affects around one in a hundred pregnant women and is often defined as persistent vomiting during pregnancy leading to weight loss of more than 15 per cent of body mass and ketosis (raised levels of ketones in the blood). HG requires hospital treatment, however if a woman who has experienced this earlier in pregnancy wants to exercise, instructors must discuss this with their primary care provider before programming any activity.

PREGNANCY AND PRE-EXISTING MEDICAL CONDITIONS

4

KEY POINTS

- Where pre-existing medical conditions are present, there may be significant risks for the pregnancy, which make activity or exercise more hazardous for the mother-to-be.
- A woman diagnosed with hypertension before pregnancy will need careful monitoring during her pregnancy to prevent complications and reduce the risk of stroke, heart problems and pre-eclampsia.
- Hypertension brought about by pregnancy (pregnancy-induced hypertension) is also a relatively common occurrence.
- An estimated 1–4 per cent of pregnant women are affected by heart problems, other than hypertension, such as congenital heart disease, rheumatic heart disease, coronary artery disease and valve disease.
- Complications associated with obesity in pregnancy include higher rates of assisted or Caesarean section deliveries, a higher rate of infection and disruption to the Caesarean incision, abnormal presentation, cervical dystocia, prolonged delivery, post-term delivery, vulvar or perineal tears, instrument delivery, induction of labour, anaesthesia problems and a longer hospital stay.
- Risks associated with obesity in pregnancy include miscarriage, gestational hypertension, pre-eclampsia, pre-gestational and gestational diabetes (GD), venous thromboembolism, preterm delivery, urinary tract infection, asthma, sleep apnoea and gallbladder disease.
- For women with diabetes who are already regular exercisers, the general consensus is that they should continue to be active, although intensity may need to be lower.
- In the exercise environment, the standard pre-exercise cautions for anyone with asthma and who is pregnant apply.
- Pregnant women with rheumatoid arthritis are unlikely to have any significant impact on the foetus as a result of the condition and being pregnant may even have a temporary beneficial effect.
- Instructors should consider and seek advice regarding other conditions such as multiple sclerosis, thyroid disease, post-partum thyroiditis, seizure disorders and disability.

CONSIDERATION OF PRE-EXISTING MEDICAL CONDITIONS

During pregnancy a woman is carrying a very precious cargo and while an otherwise healthy woman may experience side effects such as nausea, dizziness and joint discomfort, these are unlikely to have significant or serious consequences in most cases. However, there are a number of medical conditions that need consideration when working with pregnant women. Some of these may occur because of the pregnancy while others may be pre-existing conditions. However, where pre-existing medical conditions are present, there may be significant risks for the pregnancy which make activity or exercise more hazardous for the mother-to-be. In the case of any pre-existing medical condition and regardless of the current health of the woman, instructors must consult the primary antenatal care provider before recommending or commencing any form of structured activity.

CARDIOVASCULAR CONDITIONS
Hypertension

Blood pressure can be described simply as the pressure of the blood on the walls of the arteries. Measurements are recorded using two figures, systolic (maximum pressure occurring during the heartbeat), and diastolic (lowest pressure, occurring between heartbeats), with the systolic figure always given first. A healthy blood pressure in adults is considered to be around 120/80mmHg (this unit is millimetres of mercury) and below 140/90mmHg is considered normal in pregnancy. The box opposite shows the ranges of blood pressure classification in pregnant women (NICE 2010).

Blood pressure classification ranges during pregnancy (NICE 2010)

- Mildly high blood pressure between 140/90 and 149/99mmHg.
- Moderately high blood pressure between 150/100 and 159/109mmHg.
- Severely high blood pressure 160/110mmHg or higher.

Pre-existing chronic/essential hypertension

A woman diagnosed with hypertension before pregnancy will need careful monitoring during her pregnancy to prevent complications and reduce the risk of stroke, heart problems and pre-eclampsia. Instructors planning to work with such women must discuss any activity with the antenatal care provider before undertaking any form of exercise.

Gestational/pregnancy induced hypertension (PIH)

Also known as 'gestational hypertension', pregnancy-induced hypertension (PIH) is relatively common in pregnancy, usually occurring in a mild form at or close to full-term and is associated with minimal maternal or foetal complications. Mild hypertension will require ongoing monitoring by the antenatal care providers, however appropriate prescribed exercise activity is recommended to help manage the condition. If the condition worsens, particularly before 35 weeks gestation, it carries a significant risk of maternal and foetal complications so activity will probably need to cease. Instructors should always be guided by the antenatal care provider in such instances.

Table 4.1	Activity guidelines for hypertension during pregnancy
Frequency	At least five times a week
Intensity	RPE 3–5 (1–10 scale) RPE 12–14 (6–20 scale)
Time	Warm-up: At least 20 minutes Cool down: At least 12–15 minutes Main activity: As tolerated
Type	Walking, chair-based aerobics, low-intensity/impact aerobics
Additional comments	• Include pelvic floor strengthening exercises • Avoid isometric, high-resistance, high-intensity activity

For both hypertension conditions, activity guidelines for hypertension with additional pregnancy guidelines (see table 4.1) should be followed such as those adapted from the American College of Sports Medicine (ACSM).

Pre-eclampsia

Pre-eclampsia is a very serious medical condition occurring in pregnancy and almost all women who develop this will be admitted to hospital, as it may come on very suddenly and can be fatal. Pre-eclampsia can affect organs, including the heart, liver, kidneys and the brain. In severe cases it can lead to eclampsia, a type of seizure occurring in pregnancy.

If a pregnant client complains or is concerned about any of the following symptoms then it is important to advise them to contact their midwife or care provider as soon as possible (without scaring them!).

• Hypertension
• Proteinuria (protein in the urine, usually detected using a dipstick test of a urine sample. This is done routinely during antenatal visits.)

• Severe headache or migraine
• Visual disturbance
• Upper abdominal pain
• Vomiting
• Sudden onset or worsening of oedema (swelling) of the face, hands or feet
• Decreased foetal movement
• Feeling generally 'off colour'.

Heart disease

An estimated 1–4 per cent of pregnant women are affected by heart problems, other than hypertension, such as congenital heart disease, rheumatic heart disease, coronary artery disease and valve disease.

Caution

It cannot be emphasised strongly enough that any pregnant woman who indicates a history of any type of heart disease should not exercise unless the instructor has spoken directly to the antenatal care provider and received written consent to activity, as the risk of a cardiac event is significant.

Obesity

Rates of obesity are increasing and in 2010, roughly 26 per cent of all women in the general population in the UK were classed as obese. See table 4.2 for classifications according to the World Health Organization (WHO). Rates of obesity in pregnant women are of significant concern as the associated risks carry implications for maternal and foetal health. For this reason it is strongly recommended that an obese pregnant woman should exercise only with the consent of her main antenatal care provider.

Complications associated with obesity in pregnancy include higher rates of assisted or Caesarean section deliveries, a higher rate of infection and disruption to the Caesarean incision. Macrosomia (excessive birth weight of newborn baby) is becoming more common and is, along with diabetes, associated with shoulder dystocia, which is a serious and unpredictable situation where one of the baby's shoulders becomes stuck behind the pubic bone causing delay in the birth of the baby. PIH and pre-eclampsia are also more common in obese pregnant women which is why they tend to be more closely monitored in the second half of

pregnancy. The risk of developing PIH or pre-eclampsia is considered to be about 2.5 times greater for obese women and 3.2 times greater for those classified with obesity III, with the risk of pre-eclampsia being 1.6 and 3.3 times greater respectively. It has also been shown that obesity during pregnancy increases the risk of gestational diabetes (GD) by a factor of 2.6 for obese women and a factor of 4 for those with obesity III. It is further estimated that for between 5 and 10 per cent of women who develop GD, the condition will remain after delivery.

Research has also shown that the longer term consequences of obesity in pregnancy include early neonatal death and issues with weight in adolescence and adulthood, with the likelihood of being overweight as a child increasing by three times if the mother is overweight (Hemant et al 2008).

Instructors should be aware of the suggested weight gains for overweight and obese women (all classes of obesity) during pregnancy as discussed previously on page 24. Generally speaking this is between 15 and 25lbs for a mother-to-be who is overweight and up to a maximum of 14lbs for a mother-to-be who is obese according to Medforth (or between 11 and 20lbs according to the Institute of Medicine 2009). Although the risks associated with being overweight or obese during pregnancy are many and complex, table 4.3 summarises the main risks for the mother and the foetus.

Provided medical consent has been given, it is beneficial for obese pregnant women to include some activity in their daily lives. This can include walking, swimming, chair-based aerobics or any gentle activity. Table 4.4 shows exercise guidelines related to obese women who are pregnant and has been adapted from the ACSM.

Table 4.2	BMI classification (WHO)
Classification	**BMI (kg/m²)**
Underweight	< 18.4
Normal	18.5–24.9
Overweight	25–29.9
Obesity I	30–34.9
Obesity II	35–39.9
Obesity III	≥ 40

Table 4.3	Summary of associated risks of obesity in pregnancy
Mother	**Foetus**
Early pregnancy	
Miscarriage	Foetal abnormalities, neural tube defects, spina bifida, heart defects
Mid-to-late pregnancy	
Gestational hypertension, pre-eclampsia, pregestational and gestational diabetes, venous thromboembolism, preterm delivery, urinary tract infection, asthma, sleep apnoea, gallbladder disease	Foetal distress, small foetus, large foetus, stillbirth
Delivery	
Abnormal presentation, cervical dystocia+, prolonged delivery, post-term delivery, vulvar or perineal tears, instrument delivery, lower segment Caesarean section, induction of labour, anaesthesia problems, longer hospital stay	Perinatal morbidity/mortality, birth injuries, omphalocele*, macrosomia**
Postnatal	
Postpartum haemorrhage, infection, delayed healing	Brain damage, breathing problems, learning problems, susceptible to infection

+ Cervical dystocia: Failure of cervix to dilate during labour
* Omphalocele: Incomplete closure or defect of muscles of abdominal wall leading to protrusion of intestines into the umbilical cord
** Macrosomia: Excessive birth weight of newborn baby

Table 4.4	ACSM exercise guidelines for pregnant obese women

Activity guidelines for obese pregnant women

Frequency	• Start with 3 days per week with a rest day in between • Build up to 4 days per week as tolerated	
Intensity	110–131bpm (20–29 yrs) 108–127bpm (30–39 yrs)	RPE 12–14 (6–20 scale) RPE 3–5 (1–10 scale)
Time	Start at 15 minutes per session and build up to 30 minutes or as tolerated	
Type	Walking, aqua aerobics, swimming, chair-based aerobics	
Additional comments	• Include at least 5–10 minute warm-up and 5–10 minute cool down • Include pelvic floor exercises • Include muscle endurance exercises with caution	

Diabetes

As with obesity, the rates of diabetes in the UK are rising quite considerably. Diabetes is a metabolic condition where there is an absence or insufficiency of insulin production as explained previously in this book. Regardless of whether the woman has type 1, type 2 or gestational diabetes, it has been suggested by Ceysens in his 2006 review that there is insufficient information available to recommend or advise against diabetic pregnant women enrolling on exercise programmes. However, this does not mean that exercise is contraindicated. As previously discussed, pregnancy is considered to be what is known as 'diabetogenic', in that it can cause the onset of diabetes. However, appropriate physical activity and exercise are recommended to help manage the condition so women who are already regular exercisers should continue to be active, although intensity may need to be lower.

For women who were inactive prior to pregnancy, a gradual, low-intensity programme is recommended and sources such as Diabetes UK and the American Diabetes Association recommend gentle exercise of low to moderate intensity during pregnancy. Walking, cycling and swimming are considered to be ideal activities for the diabetic pregnant woman.

Foot care is also particularly important during pregnancy and caution should be observed with all forms of stretching due both to the effects of the hormone relaxin and to possible sensory neuropathy (damage to the nervous system) occurring, which may lead to unnoticed overstretching and muscle and nerve tissue damage.

Women with type 1 diabetes (which requires regular insulin injections) will need extra care during pregnancy due to the additional risks of this particular type of diabetes. For these reasons it is strongly advised that participation in activity is deferred until written consent from the primary care provider is obtained.

RESPIRATORY CONDITIONS

Shortness of breath is a normal effect of pregnancy, however if a pre-existing respiratory disorder is present there are additional factors to consider when planning exercise.

Asthma is a relatively common condition that is commonly brought on by exercise. If a client has been diagnosed as having asthma (or any other respiratory disorder such as bronchitis) then the instructor should seek guidance from the antenatal care provider if they are in any way unsure about how to progress. In the exercise environment the standard pre-exercise cautions for any person with asthma apply, such as the following:

- The woman should not undertake exercise if she does not have her inhaler with her.
- Include a longer, gradually progressed warm-up of around 15 minutes.
- Advise on an interval activity up to a maximum RPE level of 13 (on the 6–20 scale).
- Use a longer cool down including some breathing exercises or relaxation.

AUTOIMMUNE CONDITIONS

There are a number of autoimmune conditions that may pre-exist pregnancy and it is recommended that any woman with rheumatoid arthritis, lupus, multiple sclerosis or any other condition should delay becoming active in pregnancy until the instructor has spoken to the main antenatal care provider. Women with an autoimmune condition who are already active will also need specific clearance from their midwife, GP or obstetrician when they are pregnant.

Rheumatoid arthritis (RA)

Rheumatoid arthritis is an autoimmune disease that affects almost half a million people in the UK. It is generally stated that it is about three times more likely to occur in women than it is in men and the average age of onset is between 40 and 60 years and it can occur in women who are pregnant. RA is unlikely to have a significant impact on the foetus and being pregnant may even have a temporary, beneficial effect on the condition, as up to three-quarters of women find their RA symptoms are reduced in the second trimester, possibly due to hormonal changes in pregnancy.

As a note of caution, certain medications used to treat RA are not suitable for pregnancy so instructors will need to work with the antenatal care provider and the client to determine what effects this will have. Guidelines for rheumatoid arthritis include the following:

- Introduce a longer, gradually progressed warm-up with a mix of mobility and pulse raising moves.
- Low or non-impact cardiovascular training is recommended.
- Include resistance exercises that focus on endurance, low resistance and medium to high repetitions.
- Stretching needs to be carried out cautiously to avoid damage to joints, particularly those with arthritic damage.

Note: If the hips and back are affected by RA there may be issues with labour so mobility is an important part of any exercise programme.

Multiple sclerosis (MS)

Multiple sclerosis is an autoimmune condition that affects the central nervous system. Common symptoms of the condition include fatigue, visual disturbance, loss of balance and muscle control, muscle tremors, spasticity and bladder and/or bowel problems. The condition is characterised by relapses (worsening of the condition) and remission (absence or amelioration of symptoms).

MS does not appear to have any significant impact on pregnancy and may even have a protective effect, particularly in the third trimester. However, fatigue and balance issues that become worse during pregnancy may be exacerbated by MS, and bladder problems may be worsened due to the weight of the growing foetus on the bladder. Any planned exercise programme should take these factors into account by reducing intensity, shortening the length of the session and doing cardiovascular and muscle endurance work on alternate days to avoid fatigue. Following birth, there is a risk of relapse as hormone levels return to normal.

With this particular condition an instructor should have the knowledge (and qualification) relating to the condition or should otherwise seek advice from the antenatal care provider.

Thyroid disease

Thyroid conditions in pregnancy can lead to significant complications and have an impact on the health of the mother and foetus. For this reason, it is strongly recommended that instructors seek advice from the antenatal care provider before exercise is undertaken.

Post-partum thyroiditis

This condition develops after birth and usually resolves quickly. However, in some cases it can become longer term hypothyroidism, which will need treatment.

SEIZURE DISORDERS

Seizure disorders such as epilepsy carry a higher risk of birth defects so for this reason it is strongly recommended that instructors seek advice from the antenatal care provider before exercise is undertaken.

DISABILITY

Exercise is an important factor in functional ability for women with disabilities and during pregnancy, provided the disability is accommodated, physical activity is just as important as for non-disabled women.

EXERCISE DURING IN VITRO FERTILISATION (IVF) PREGNANCY

Once an in vitro fertilisation (IVF) pregnancy is established, it is considered appropriate for the woman to participate in activity according to the recommended guidelines. However, if the pregnancy is the result of IVF it is quite common to find that the mother does not want to do any activity that she feels may jeopardise the pregnancy. Although appropriate activity is unlikely to affect the pregnancy, from a psychological perspective it is better to be guided by the woman's feelings at this time.

EXERCISE FOLLOWING A FAILED PREGNANCY

It is important to recognise that not all pregnancies conclude with a live birth. Sadly some pregnancies end in miscarriage, termination or a stillbirth. Ectopic pregnancy, where the fertilised egg implants outside the uterus, often in the fallopian tube, is another cause of failed pregnancy. An ectopic pregnancy is likely to be surgically terminated as if left to develop it could cause the fallopian tube to rupture, leading to haemorrhage and potentially serious consequences for the mother. In such cases the woman is likely to be receiving appropriate care to ensure her physical and psychological health are looked after, however, the physical effects of pregnancy do need to be considered if and when she returns to exercise.

Relaxin will remain in the body for several months so joints are likely to be less stable meaning care should be taken when stretching. Breast enlargement, tenderness and milk production may remain for a period which can affect comfort or position of exercises. There may be weight gain associated with the pregnancy that the client wants to get rid of as quickly as possible to remove any upsetting reminders, which can lead to overexercising. Additionally, a subsequent pregnancy may result in the woman being reluctant to be active 'just in case'. Although it is not likely to have an effect or cause a miscarriage, her feelings are paramount and an instructor should accept that.

PSYCHOLOGICAL IMPLICATIONS OF PREGNANCY

5

KEY POINTS

- Mental health conditions can occur as a result of pregnancy and it is also possible for there to be pre-existing conditions that may be exacerbated during pregnancy.
- Common mental health issues in pregnancy include those such as anxiety, stress, panic disorder, obsessive compulsive disorder (OCD), phobias and depression.
- Mild to moderate forms of these conditions are likely to be treated in primary care unless the condition becomes severe when the woman may be treated in secondary care such as in hospital or under the supervision of the community mental health team.
- Other severe and enduring conditions such as schizophrenia, bipolar disorder, psychosis, eating disorders or substance misuse will be treated in specialist environments.
- The key symptoms of anxiety and stress during pregnancy include dizziness, increased heart rate, palpitations, shallower breathing, increased sweating, headaches, tremors, muscle tension, chest or stomach pain, excessive worry, inability to concentrate, catastrophising, negative thinking, insomnia or hypersomnia, increased or decreased eating, smoking, social withdrawal, development of phobias and panic attacks.
- The fear of panic attacks can sometimes lead to the development of a condition known as agoraphobia, which is characterised by a fear of being in a place from which it is difficult to escape.
- It is thought that OCD may be triggered by pregnancy, perhaps due to a need for cleanliness and safety, or because of the fear of causing harm to the foetus during pregnancy or to the baby.
- It is estimated that almost one in three pregnant women experience some type of depression.
- There is a wealth of evidence for the efficacy of activity and exercise in improving mental health and, specifically, for preventing or alleviating depression and anxiety in the general population and it is thought that this will also occur during pregnancy.

CONSIDERATION OF PSYCHOLOGICAL CHANGES

As already discussed, pregnancy is a time of many physiological changes, however, the emotional and psychological changes that also occur can have a significant impact on the well-being of the mother and baby. While this means that mental health conditions can occur as a result of pregnancy, it is also possible for there to be pre-existing conditions that may be exacerbated as a result of the pregnancy.

Common mental health issues reported in pregnancy include those such as anxiety, stress, panic disorder, obsessive compulsive disorder (OCD), phobias and depression. Mild to moderate forms of these conditions are more likely to be treated in primary care unless the condition becomes severe, whereupon the woman may be treated in a secondary care environment such as in hospital or under the supervision of the community mental health team. More severe and enduring conditions such as schizophrenia, bipolar disorder, psychosis, eating disorders or substance misuse will most likely be treated in specialist environments and any instructor who is working with a client who discloses a particular severe condition should contact the specialist psychiatric or antenatal care provider as soon as possible as there may be negative consequences as a result of undertaking an exercise programme with such a condition.

Anecdotally, there appears to be common concern that pregnancy will affect the mother psychologically as well as physiologically, although the concerns tend to change from ante- to post-natal stages. For example, some of the more common psychological effects in the early stages of pregnancy include over-reacting to minor situations and being prone to mood swings as well as losing self-esteem because of concern over bodily changes (such as an increase in weight and, in fewer cases, varicose veins). As the pregnancy goes on into the later stages there are often concerns over the ability to cope and feelings of being anxious about the delivery.

Even though the area of mental health is vast and further reading is always recommended, there are commonly associated psychological areas that the instructor should familiarise themselves with.

ANXIETY AND STRESS

The effects of anxiety can have a negative impact on pregnancy although the specific cause or link is still not fully understood. These negative effects can include placental abruption (separation of the placenta from the uterine wall prior to delivery), although this is rare as it only affects about 1 per cent of pregnancies, preterm labour, a low APGAR score (see appendix 2, page 173) and low birth weight. Anxiety may also occur due to concerns about lifestyle behaviours that occurred between conception and finding out about the pregnancy such as drinking or smoking. It is important however to distinguish between anxiety that occurs due to 'normal' pregnancy concerns and pathological anxiety that may need specialist treatment.

It is widely acknowledged that many pregnant women find they become anxious about a variety of issues relating to pregnancy, birth and bringing up children, so much so that anxiety may be considered a 'normal' effect of pregnancy and beyond offering reassurance, support and a willing ear, does not usually need treatment. However, pathological anxiety is a more serious concern as the physiological and psychological effects combined can usually have a negative effect on the well-being of the mother and the foetus.

Table 5.1	Key symptoms of anxiety and stress	
Physical/autonomic	**Mental**	**Behavioural**
Dizziness	Gratuitous or excessive worry	Insomnia or hypersomnia
Increased heart rate*	Inability to concentrate	Increased or decreased eating
Palpitations	Catastrophising	Smoking
Faster, shallower breathing*	Negative thinking	Social withdrawal
Increased sweating*	Tension	Development of phobias
Headaches	Unable to 'switch off'	Panic attacks
Tremors		
Muscle tension*		
Unable to relax		
Chest or stomach pain		

* *Note:* These are also physiological responses to activity so it is important to explain that these may occur to prevent an increase in anxiety levels during exercise.

Some key symptoms of anxiety and stress that are commonly cited are shown in table 5.1. However, as many of these are common to pregnancy as well, it may be difficult to determine if the symptoms are due to the effects of pregnancy or to a deeper or pre-existing mental health issue. It should also be noted that during pregnancy, anxiety may lead to the development of other mental health issues such as panic disorder, phobias or OCD. Exercise guidelines are available for stress-related conditions during pregnancy such as those in table 5.2, adapted from the American College of Sports Medicine (ACSM).

PANIC DISORDER AND PHOBIA

Although this may appear a very general sounding condition, panic disorder is often described as being characterised by episodes, or attacks, of severe anxiety leading to extreme forms of the symptoms that are listed in table 5.1. The fear of these panic attacks can sometimes lead to the development of a condition which is known as 'agoraphobia'. This condition is typically characterised by a fear of being in a place from which it is difficult to escape or in which a person feels unsafe. If this is the case it may cause the mother-to-be to feel reluctant to go out unless absolutely necessary, for example to attend antenatal appointments, and can result in her becoming socially withdrawn.

OBSESSIVE COMPULSIVE DISORDER (OCD)

Obsessive compulsive disorder is characterised by rituals or habits that need to be performed in a specific order or a set number of times. The more common compulsions are repetitive behaviours like checking, ordering, washing or cleaning, and

Table 5.2	Activity guidelines for stress and anxiety disorder		
	Cardiovascular	**Strength**	**Flexibility**
Frequency	3–5 days a week	2 days per week	After each session
Intensity	50%–85% MHR	60–85% 1RM	Stretch to point of tightness, avoid discomfort
Time	20–30 minutes	1 set of 8–12 reps	15–30 secs per stretch
Type	Walking, jogging, cycling, low intensity/impact	Resistance machine, body weight, free weights, etc.	
Additional comments	• Warm up and cool down before and after each session for at least 5–10 minutes per session. • Be aware that the physiological response to activity may mimic the anxiety or stress response. Tell the client what they may experience as they start to exercise to ensure they do not think they are having an anxiety attack.		

a fear of contamination which can have a minor or major effect on everyday life and activities. Obsessions can include unwanted or repulsive thoughts that the person feels they cannot control. Ritualised patterns of behaviour may occur to compensate for or distract from these thoughts.

It is suggested that OCD may be triggered by pregnancy, perhaps due to a need for cleanliness and safety, or because of fears of causing harm to the foetus during pregnancy or to the baby following delivery (Kalra et al 2005). This in turn may lead to reluctance to participate in any form of exercise or activity for fear of harming the foetus in some way, therefore, undue pressure to be active may cause considerable and distressing anxiety and the wishes or feelings of the mother-to-be must always be a priority for an instructor.

DEPRESSION

It is estimated that almost one in three pregnant women experience some type of depression (Price 2007). In another study by Evans et al in 2001 it was suggested that levels may actually be higher in the antenatal period than the postnatal period.

One of the major issues for women who experience antenatal depression is a reluctance to admit it at a time when they are generally assumed to be 'on top of the world' which means many cases may be undiagnosed and therefore untreated, increasing the risk of postnatal or clinical depression after delivery.

Although the symptoms of depression are numerous, the key symptoms which have been adapted from the American Psychiatric Association (2000) include the following, of which five or more should be present nearly every day over a two-week period for a diagnosis to be made.

- Depressed mood
- Significantly reduced interest in previously pleasurable activities
- Weight loss or gain when not dieting

- Insomnia or hypersomnia
- Slowed down or agitated movement patterns
- Fatigue and/or loss of energy
- Feelings of worthlessness, pointlessness or guilt
- Unable to concentrate or think
- Thoughts of death or suicide (Note: there may be no intention to commit suicide).

There are a number of factors that may increase the risk of depression occurring in pregnancy. These factors can be classified in different ways but according to sources such as Leigh and Milgron in 2008 and Lee et al in 2007, risk factors for depression should be classified under the headings of medical and chemical, emotional and socio-economic factors, as summarised in table 5.3. As is the case with risk factors related to any other condition, this does not mean that depression is going to occur, it merely means that there is a greater risk than if no risk factors were present.

Table 5.3	Risk factors for antenatal depression	
Medical/chemical	**Emotional**	**Other**
Increased pregnancy hormones	Anxiety about pregnancy	Young age
Neurotransmitter imbalance	History of miscarriage or termination	Low educational achievement
Past history of depression	Unwanted pregnancy	Low income
Family history of depression	Fears about the future	History of childhood abuse
	Body image issues	History of drinking
	Low self-esteem	

Table 5.4	Activity guidelines for mental health conditions		
	Cardiovascular	**Strength**	**Flexibility**
Frequency	At least 4 days a week	2 days per week	5 days per week
Intensity	RPE 3–5 (1–10 scale) RPE 11–14 (6–20 scale)	50–70% 1RM	Maintain stretch below discomfort point
Time	20–30 minutes	1 set of 8–12 reps	20–60 seconds per stretch
Type	Walking, chair-based aerobics, low-intensity/low-impact aerobics, swimming	Resistance machines, body weight, free weights, etc.	
Additional comments	• Warm up and cool down before and after each session • At least 5–10 minutes per session		

There is a wealth of evidence for the efficacy of activity and exercise in improving mental health and, specifically, for preventing or alleviating depression and anxiety in the general population. Although the role of exercise in preventing or alleviating antenatal depression has not been researched in as much depth, it is likely that these benefits will occur, making appropriate exercise important in pregnancy. It is important to ensure that any exercise advice does not contribute to or exacerbate anxiety or depression so an emphasis on what the mother-to-be enjoys and feels comfortable with is important. Table 5.4 shows suggested activity guidelines adapted from the ACSM.

PREGNANCY AND SEVERE AND ENDURING MENTAL HEALTH CONDITIONS

Severe and enduring mental health conditions include schizophrenia, bipolar disorder, psychosis, personality disorders and severe depression. A woman who has a pre-existing condition that may be exacerbated by pregnancy, or who develops a severe or major mental health condition during pregnancy is likely to be in the care of secondary mental health care services and have a designated care co-ordinator as well as an antenatal care provider. In such cases, an instructor must work with the whole team of care providers and it is essential to maintain up-to-date and accurate records and to provide regular feedback to this team.

PREGNANCY AND ACTIVITY

6

KEY POINTS

- There are two main bodies that recommend exercise during pregnancy; the Royal College of Obstetricians and Gynaecologists (RCOG) and the American Congress of Obstetricians and Gynecologists (ACOG).
- The benefits to the mother of doing regular physical activity during the first trimester include reduced or alleviated symptoms of pregnancy, improved social aspects, maintaining bone density throughout and a decreased risk of diabetes.
- The benefits to the mother of doing regular physical activity during the second trimester include increased energy levels and reserve, improved digestion, reduced weight gain (fat), reduced back pain and enhanced maternal well-being.
- The benefits to the mother of doing regular physical activity during the third trimester include increased self-esteem, better posture, improved sleep, greater energy levels and shorter and easier labour.
- The postnatal benefits to the mother of doing regular physical activity during pregnancy include a leaner baby, a quicker return to pre-pregnancy weight and fitness, reduced bone loss and reduced depression.
- It is thought that foetal stress levels are lower in women who exercised throughout pregnancy.
- Some of the risks of exercising during pregnancy include joint injury, hyperthermia, increased risk of a miscarriage, reduced blood flow and oxygen delivery, hypotension, umbilical cord problems, waters can break, extended or difficult labour and poor breast milk, therefore it is important that instructors always follow published exercise guidelines.

BENEFITS OF PHYSICAL ACTIVITY

Instructors are usually somewhat hesitant (and justifiably so) when it comes to giving exercise advice to pregnant women, therefore, in relation to advice and guidelines for exercise and pregnancy, there are two main bodies that are recommended by the authors; they are the Royal College of Obstetricians and Gynaecologists (RCOG) and the American Congress of Obstetricians and Gynecologists (ACOG)

(ACOG). Both of these bodies agree that physical activity during an uncomplicated pregnancy should be actively recommended for the purpose of a potential host of maternal and foetal benefits.

While it is potentially difficult to study the effects of exercise during pregnancy on the mother-to-be and foetus (for obvious ethical reasons), there is however a substantial amount of research evidence that has been carried out relating to the effects on the mother-to-be, but there is not as much evidence in terms of the beneficial effects to the foetus.

BENEFITS TO THE MOTHER

The benefits to both the mother and mother-to-be of doing regular physical activity leading up to and during pregnancy can be slightly different depending on the trimester and postnatal period, as can be seen in table 6.1. The summary outlines some of the main reported potential benefits which have been adapted from the RCOG and the ACOG.

Reduced pregnancy symptoms

It is often demonstrated by way of research studies that many of the symptoms of pregnancy are either

Try this!

Think of as many benefits to mother and baby that can be gained by exercising before and during pregnancy. This could be either physiological or psychological.

reduced or alleviated in women who have followed a regular exercise programme leading up to and throughout the duration of the pregnancy. These effects appear to be greater in the 1st trimester but can carry on into the 2nd and 3rd trimesters.

Social aspect

By encouraging mothers-to-be to take part in exercise, they will often get the opportunity to meet other mothers-to-be and share experiences. This may help to reassure them that they are not alone, and what they are going through is a natural and normal process.

Maintenance of bone density

By incorporating weight-bearing activity into the programme, bone density can be maintained

Table 6.1	Potential benefits of physical activity for pregnant women		
First trimester	**Second trimester**	**Third trimester**	**Postnatal**
Reduce or alleviate symptoms of pregnancy	Increased energy levels and reserve	Increased self-esteem	Leaner baby
Social aspects	Improved digestion	Better posture	Quicker return to pre-pregnancy weight and fitness
Maintain bone density throughout	Reduced weight gain (fat)	Improved sleep	
Decreased risk of diabetes	Reduced back pain	More energy	Reduced bone loss
	Enhanced maternal well-being	Shorter and easier labour	Reduce depression

throughout the pregnancy and afterwards, avoiding the result of calcium lost through breastfeeding.

Decreased risk of diabetes

Research from the Harvard School of Public Health (HSPH) in 2010 (published in *Diabetes Care*) reported that regular exercise before or in early pregnancy can reduce the risk of gestational diabetes by up to 55 per cent.

Greater energy levels

The smooth muscle of blood vessel walls relaxes under the influence of progesterone during pregnancy. As a result of exercising or being regularly active, blood flow can be improved and potentially reduce the formation of varicose veins and increase the supply of oxygen, which results in the feeling of increased energy levels.

Control of weight gain

A certain amount of weight gain is essential in pregnancy for different reasons such as protection and feeding of the baby. Excessive weight gain however can increase the risk of complications (see page 38) and can also exacerbate any back and joint pain already present. It is generally found that a regular exercise programme can help to control this.

Better pregnancy posture

By including specific exercises, especially for the back and abdominals, the impact of the developing pregnancy on posture can be reduced. This in turn can help to alleviate back, neck and shoulder pain.

Increased well-being and self-esteem

Pregnancy can often have a negative effect on the mother-to-be as a result of some of the changes that are happening in the body. By maintaining good posture and body awareness, regular exercise has often been demonstrated to help to improve a host of psychological factors including well-being, self-esteem, self-image and confidence.

Easier labour

Performing appropriate activity during pregnancy can help to improve fitness in preparation for childbirth. It has been shown that fitter mothers tend to cope with labour more easily.

Leaner babies

Babies born to exercising mothers tend to be of similar dimensions (length and head circumference) but have less fat on them than babies born to non-exercising mothers. This is potentially better for them as they have a healthier body composition. One study that supports this was carried out in 2010 by Hopkins and colleagues at the University of Auckland in New Zealand, which showed that women who did moderate intensity aerobic exercise five times a week had lower-weight babies than those that did no exercise. The study by Owe and colleagues in 2009 which was undertaken in Norway also supports this.

Quicker postnatal recovery

Muscles that are toned and strong prior to and during pregnancy normally recover more quickly after delivery. This could have a number of positive effects such as enabling the mother to cope with the physical demands of motherhood better and also improving psychological aspects by regaining pre-pregnancy shape more quickly. A study carried out in Melbourne, Australia (published in *Physical Therapy*, March 2010) showed that regular exercise throughout pregnancy could help postnatal mothers lower their risk of depression by up to 50 per cent.

BENEFITS TO THE BABY

As far as benefits to the foetus are concerned, research by Paisley et al (2003) has suggested that foetuses of exercising women tolerate labour better than the foetuses of non-exercising women. It has also been shown, such as in the investigation by Clapp in 2002, that foetal stress levels are lower in women who exercised throughout pregnancy (at 50 per cent of their preconception level) compared to well-conditioned athletes who discontinued exercise before the end of their first trimester.

Stress levels in the foetus were measured in several ways. One of the methods used was the APGAR test. This clinical test was developed by Virginia Apgar in 1952 and was designed to evaluate a newborn's physical condition just after birth and to determine any immediate need for extra medical or emergency care. The test is normally done twice, once at 1 minute after birth then again at 5 minutes after birth. For further information on this test see appendix 2, page 173.

RISKS ASSOCIATED WITH PHYSICAL ACTIVITY

Even though there are many benefits of a regular physical activity programme right through pregnancy and for the postnatal period (as there are with

Table 6.2	Potential risks of physical activity for pregnant women
Risk	**Explanation**
Joint injury	Particular damage to the bones in the joints which can lead to osteoarthritis.
Hyperthermia	The body temperature can rise more than it would normally and excessive temperature (no more than 39.2°C) could affect the baby's development.
Increased risk of a miscarriage	The risk of a miscarriage is obviously higher as the amount and intensity of physical activity increases particularly due to heat stress.
Blood flow and oxygen delivery is reduced	Oxygen is required to supply the working muscles doing the physical activity, which can be diverted away from the placenta.
Hypotension	When lying on the back the foetus can press on blood vessels (the vena cava in particular) causing a loss of blood pressure.
Umbilical cord problems	High-impact activities can result in the umbilical cord being wrapped around the foetus.
Waters can break	High-intensity or impact exercise can cause the waters to break.
Extended or difficult labour	If abdominal and pelvic floor muscles are too strong they can in some cases extend the labour period.
Poor breast milk	Strenuous exercise has been shown in some cases to reduce the quantity and quality of the mother's breast milk.

all populations), there are many associated risks that need to be considered. Again, even though the research information in this area is limited, a common sense approach to err on the side of caution is highly recommended. Table 6.2 outlines some of the risks to pregnant women associated with physical activity which are adapted from those published by the RCOG and the ACOG.

REDUCED JOINT STABILITY
Because of the production during pregnancy of the hormone relaxin, ligaments around the joints do not provide as much support as they normally do. Any exercise, therefore, that causes impact through the joints can increase the risk of damage to the surrounding cartilage, which may increase the risk of osteoarthritis in the longer term.

OVERHEATING
Studies on human babies and the effects of overheating (also known as hyperthermia) have not been done, however studies on rats appear to indicate that overheating can cause birth defects and miscarriage, especially in the first trimester. Having said this, during pregnancy the body becomes more efficient at keeping cooler by increasing sweating and vasodilation to the skin so heat is dissipated more effectively.

REDUCED OXYGEN TO THE PLACENTA
This is often regarded as a concern, however the placenta is extremely efficient at extracting the oxygen it needs for foetal development from the maternal circulation.

SUPINE HYPOTENSIVE SYNDROME
This is the term that is used to describe low blood pressure as a result of the mother lying on her back (supine position) mainly in the second and third trimesters. In this position the weight of the growing uterus can compress the inferior vena cava (blood vessel going to the heart), restricting the amount of blood that can be delivered. Guidelines from ACOG and other medical groups recommend that no exercises are carried out in the supine position after 16–20 weeks. Even though there is little research evidence to support this, the authors recommend erring on the side of caution and following these guidelines.

HYPOGLYCAEMIA (LOW BLOOD SUGAR)
During very prolonged activity, hypoglycaemia may be a concern, however for most activity, energy requirements are met by utilising fat as fuel, sparing carbohydrates for the foetus.

STRESS INCONTINENCE
The weight of the foetus places additional stress on the pelvic floor during pregnancy which may lead to weakness and incontinence, both during activity and when coughing, laughing or sneezing.

LOW BACK STRAIN
The additional weight of the baby and the forward shift in the centre of gravity leads to postural changes which can put strain on the lower back.

PHYSICAL ACTIVITY GUIDELINES
Any pregnant woman wishing to start a programme of regular physical activity should always obtain clearance from their doctor or physician prior to starting. Anyone wishing to supervise activity in the antenatal stage should make sure that they are qualified to do so by undertaking one of the

many courses that are available. Once individuals are qualified to supervise physical activity for this population, they should become familiar with specific written questionnaires (known as screening forms) that are used to help identify pregnancies in which the risk of abnormality is higher than usual. One such screening form is the PARmed-X for PREGNANCY (see appendix 3, page 174) which is available from the Canadian Society for Exercise Physiology (CSEP).

As far as general activity guidelines are concerned, it is suggested that if women are reasonably active prior to becoming pregnant and are generally healthy, then there should be no problems in continuing recommended activity throughout the pregnancy. However, if the individual was sedentary prior to becoming pregnant it is recommended that only low-intensity activity should be undertaken. More specific guidelines have been published by the RCOG and the ACOG, however an overview of the guidelines includes the following:

- Use the talk test or Borg Rate of Perceived Exertion (RPE) scale to determine exercise intensity.
- Do not exercise to the point of exhaustion.
- Do not exercise in the supine position (on the back) and minimise motionless standing.
- Dress in light comfortable clothing and keep well hydrated.

Try this!

See if you can write down any guidelines that you think might be related to exercise during pregnancy.

- Ingest carbohydrate (30–50g) prior to exercise.
- Avoid abdominal exercises other than transversus abdominis (TA) engagement.
- Maintain training heart rate under 140bpm.
- Avoid high-impact activities.

The ACOG/RCOG have also published information relating to certain circumstances when pregnant women should not do or should stop doing any form of physical activity. These circumstances are more commonly known as 'contraindications' to exercise. Table 6.3 lists the absolute and relative contraindications to physical activity in pregnancy and also explains related situations in which any activity that is in progress should be stopped immediately. The relative contraindications do not necessarily mean no activity can be done, but they do mean an instructor will need to get advice on the suitability of exercise from the woman's care provider, or that only medically supervised exercise should be undertaken.

Even though some of these terms may be unfamiliar, if the intention is to supervise a physical activity programme for someone who is pregnant, these questions should be asked before any activity is undertaken, particularly if they have any of the contraindications. This shouldn't be a problem as someone who is pregnant should have a good understanding of the terms and be used to answering questions. It is important also that the supervisor (or the individual) should constantly monitor the situation during all physical activity for circumstances that require the activity to be stopped immediately (as in table 6.3 as suggested by the ACOG) and in some cases to seek medical advice.

As far as general guidelines for antenatal physical activity are concerned, table 6.4 provides an overview

Table 6.3	Contraindications and reasons to stop activity for pregnant women (RCOG)

Absolute contraindications to activity

- Cardiac disease
- Restrictive lung disease
- Incompetent cervix/cerclage
- Multiple gestation at risk of preterm labour
- Persistent bleeding in the second and third trimesters
- Placenta praevia (where the placenta is partly or fully covering the cervix) after 26 weeks
- Pre-eclampsia or pregnancy-induced hypertension
- Preterm labour (previous/present)
- Preterm rupture of membranes

Relative contraindications to activity

- Severe anaemia (haemoglobin less than 100g/L)
- Unevaluated maternal cardiac arrhythmia
- Chronic bronchitis
- Poorly controlled type 1 diabetes
- Extreme morbid obesity (BMI >40)
- Extreme underweight (BMI <12)
- Extremely sedentary lifestyle
- Intrauterine growth restriction (IUGR) in current pregnancy
- Poorly controlled hypertension/pre-eclampsia
- Orthopaedic limitations
- Poorly controlled thyroid disease
- Poorly controlled seizure disorder
- Heavy smoker (more than 20 cigarettes/day)

Reasons to stop activity

- Excessive shortness of breath
- Chest pain or palpitations
- Presyncope (feeling faint or feeling about to faint) or dizziness
- Painful uterine contractions or preterm labour
- Calf pain or swelling
- Leakage of amniotic fluid
- Vaginal bleeding
- Excessive fatigue
- Abdominal pain, particularly in back or pubic area
- Pelvic girdle pain
- Reduced foetal movement
- Dyspnoea (shortness of breath) before exertion
- Headache or visual disturbance
- Muscle weakness
- Sudden calf pain or swelling in the ankles, hands or face
- Insufficient weight gain (less than 1kg per month) during last two trimesters

Table 6.4	Physical activity guidelines for antenatal women	
	Aerobic training	**Strength training**
Mode	Walking, cycling and water-based activities are good for this condition	Continue as normal if already active. If not, slow progression from body weight to machines/free weights
Intensity	• RPE level 10–14 • 60–80% HRmax	• Avoid heavy loads • Overload by increasing repetitions
Duration	• 5–45 minutes per session • Increase by 2 minutes per week but only between the 13th and 28th weeks	• Perform 1 to 3 sets of 15–20RM • 1–2 minutes' rest between exercises
Frequency	Active person: • 3–4 per week up to 14th week • 3–5 per week up to 28th week • 3 per week after 28th week Non-active person: • None before 13th week • 3 per week 13th–36th weeks • 1–2 per week after 36th week	• 2–3 sessions per week • Encourage other forms of exercise • Decrease weight and sets and increase recovery time as pregnancy progresses
Precautions	• Avoid high-impact activities and excessive repetition • Watch for signs of overheating	• If no experience prior to pregnancy, do not start • Avoid overstretching and overhead lifts

General precautions:

• Non-active women are advised to seek medical approval **before** beginning a programme of activity.

• If any activity causes pain or discomfort it should be stopped immediately.

• Do the rectus abdominis check 6–12 weeks after delivery (see page 168) before doing certain abdominal exercises.

• Be aware of episiotomy and take appropriate steps.

• Avoid motionless standing.

• Avoid supine exercises (lying on the back) after 16 weeks.

taken from a variety of sources such as the RCOG, the ACOG and the American College of Sports Medicine (ACSM). Note that activity should only be progressed between the 13th and 28th weeks.

Did you know?

The uterus is one of the very few muscles in the body that can contract and then relax in a contracted state.

LABOUR AND DELIVERY

It is not the intention of this book to discuss labour or delivery in any detail, however it is useful for instructors to understand the types of delivery so they can advise clients on when it is appropriate to resume activity. There are three methods of delivery:

NORMAL VAGINAL DELIVERY

A normal vaginal delivery is often referred to as being in labour and this consists of three stages. During the first stage the cervix dilates (widens) to approximately 10cm in preparation for the birth of the baby. Uterine contractions occur during the first stage and cause dilation of the cervix and these can be extremely painful! This stage lasts an average of 12–18 hours for a first delivery and 7 hours for second and subsequent deliveries. The second stage is the actual birth of the baby and lasts an average of 1–2 hours for first babies, 15–45 minutes subsequently. During this stage the baby travels down the birth canal and the head, then shoulders and body are delivered. The third stage of labour is the delivery of the placenta which occurs up to 15 minutes after the baby has been delivered.

ASSISTED VAGINAL DELIVERY

This is similar to a normal delivery however during the second stage assistance in the form of a ventouse cap (a vacuum extractor) or, less commonly nowadays, forceps (pincer-like instruments designed to fit round the head of the baby) are used to facilitate the birth. An episiotomy (incision into vaginal/

perineal tissues) may be done to widen the passage and also to minimise the risk of additional tearing. If an episiotomy or tear occurs then stitches will be applied to help keep correct alignment during healing. These can be very uncomfortable and can lead to reluctance to place any pressure on the genital region for some weeks to come.

CAESAREAN SECTION

This is an operation performed to deliver the baby through the abdominal wall. The majority of Caesareans are lower uterine segment Caesarean sections (LUSCS) where a transverse incision is made low down in the uterus. An emergency Caesarean section may be performed if the mother or baby become distressed during delivery or it may be planned (elective) in advance in certain circumstances, for example due to the position of the baby (breech or transverse position), or if the placenta is lying over the lower part of the uterus (placenta praevia). The Caesarean section incision needs care afterwards as it can become infected which will delay any return to activity.

Most new mothers will attend a six-week post-natal check to see how recovery is progressing and ensure that they are ready to return to normal activities, including exercise. In the immediate postnatal period before this check, only gentle walking or physiotherapy recommended exercises should be carried out.

2

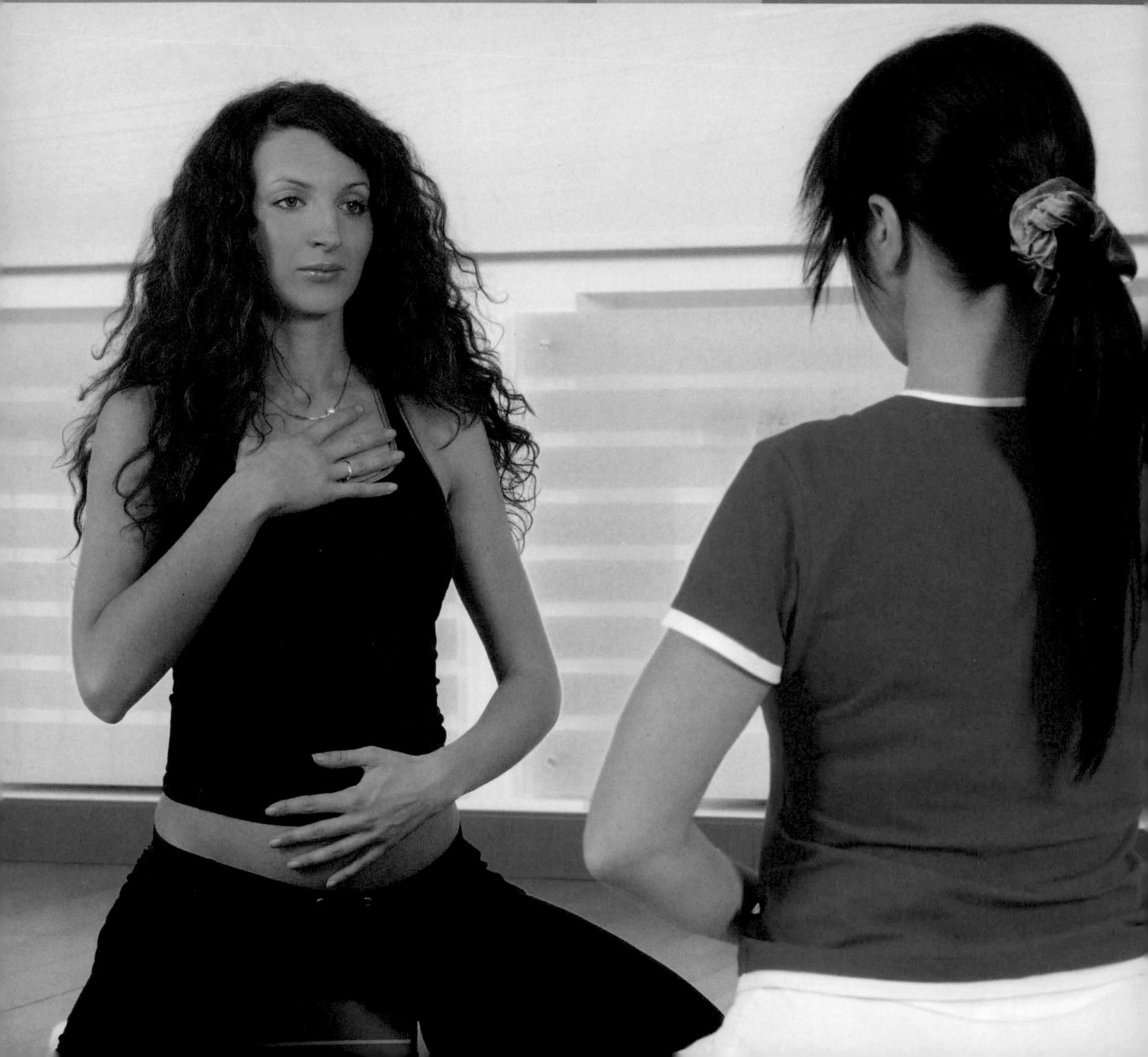

PART **TWO**

PREPARATION

BEHAVIOUR // CHANGE

7

KEY POINTS

- Many surveys show that much of the adult population does not engage in any form of regular exercise.
- Getting an individual to partake in a regular exercise programme is referred to as 'behavioural change'.
- The Transtheoretical Model of Stages of Change that was first designed by Prochaska and DiClemente was originally developed to help people stop smoking.
- Approximately 15 per cent of all individuals will experience relapse when trying to maintain a programme of regular exercise.
- There are various strategies that can be used to help an individual through the discrete stages of change.
- There are four broad exercise categories associated with pregnant women: currently inactive, currently active for health, currently active and active athlete.
- For women who decide to exercise to avoid gaining weight, careful management must be employed to avoid over-exercising and risking negative effects to the foetus.
- Many people become regularly active in order to prevent or reduce the effects of medical conditions such as heart disease, diabetes, obesity, arthritis and asthma.
- An instructor has a duty of care to ensure that any pregnant client with whom they are working is training at an appropriate level to minimise the risk of potential problems with the pregnancy.
- Pregnancy is not the time to try to improve fitness. Instructors should encourage pregnant athletes to just maintain a reasonable level of fitness.

STAGES OF CHANGE

It is not surprising to learn that much of the adult population does not engage in any form of regular exercise let alone follow a specific programme. Therefore, to be successful in getting an individual to partake in a regular exercise programme often requires a substantial change in lifestyle and habits. Any type of change relating to this should be more accurately referred to as 'behavioural change'. It can be extremely challenging for both the individual and the instructor to overcome sedentary habits that may have been in place for many years. Research has confirmed this as it is generally accepted that behavioural change is typically a long-term process so the nine months of pregnancy may not be long enough to see major changes in lifestyle or habit.

Scientists have studied behavioural change for many years and accepted models such as that proposed by researchers Prochaska and DiClemente (Transtheoretical Model of Stages of Change) have been developed to help the instructor facilitate the process of making sustainable changes in behaviour for their clients. The Stages of Change model, as can be seen in figure 7.1, proposes that there are a number of discrete stages in relation to making any type of lifestyle change such as smoking cessation or alcohol rehabilitation. Indeed, the research carried out by Prochaska and DiClemente used smoking cessation as the theme for the conception of the model,

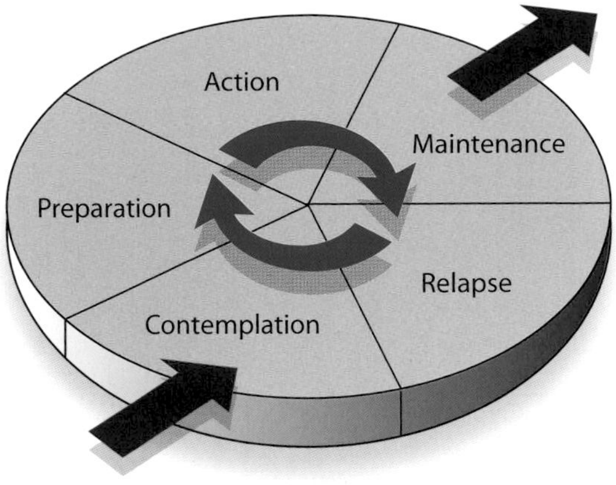

Figure 7.1 Stages of Change model

however, this model can be applied to exercise uptake and is the one most commonly used in the health and fitness industry.

Table 7.1	Discrete stages in the Stages of Change model
Stage	**Description**
Pre-contemplation (I won't)	This is where the individual does not intend to take any action in the short term (usually within about six months).
Contemplation (I might)	This is where the individual intends to take action soon but is unsure about the change.
Preparation (I will)	The individual has taken steps towards some kind of action, such as taking out a gym membership, and is planning to act (normally within one month).
Action (I am)	This is where the individual has taken some kind of action and changed their behaviour in the short term.
Maintenance (I have)	This is a period of behavioural change lasting for more than six months and with a firm commitment to the particular change.
Relapse	This is where individuals can completely drop out and discontinue any form of exercise. This can happen at any stage and many times over.

As can be seen from the exercise-related Stages of Change model there are several stages which can vary in duration depending on the particular individual. The reason the model is cyclical in nature is that an individual can start at any point on the circle and can also drop out or relapse at any stage. Also, an individual can go from one stage to the next and back again without ever moving any further in the stage model. It is widely known that approximately 15 per cent of all individuals will experience relapse back to the contemplation or precontemplation stage. In the adapted Prochaska and DiClemente model the stages of change have been described in table 7.1 in relation to exercise.

Depending on the stage at which an individual might be, the instructor can use various strategies to help the individual through the stages of change with a view to helping them to reach the maintenance stage, even though instructors should be aware of and focus on the move from the contemplation stage to the action stage, as this is often reported to be the most difficult transition. Strategies such as 'cognitive' and 'behavioural' processes are sometimes used to help clients move from one stage to the next, however these psychological strategies extend beyond the scope of this book, therefore, instructors and individuals are encouraged to increase their knowledge of this particular area

as part of self-development and progression. It should be emphasised however, that the Stages of Change model should ideally be used with clients who are contemplating pregnancy. If this is the case it would be ideal for an individual to have reached the maintenance stage before they conceive.

EXERCISE CATEGORIES

Participating in a programme of regular exercise is difficult enough for most people and when the effects of pregnancy such as tiredness, anxiety, breathlessness and other symptoms are added it can be very hard for a non-exerciser to find the motivation to become active. In terms of the type of pregnant women that an instructor may come across, there are four broad exercise categories as shown in figure 7.2.

Currently inactive

Many inactive women often feel that they should start to do some sort of activity during their pregnancy in order to benefit both their health and the health of the baby during and after pregnancy. However, it is important to find out the reasons why a woman in this category would want to start exercising as this is likely to determine the level of motivation and predict adherence. This will help in devising a realistic and effective programme of exercise and activity that the client feels is both

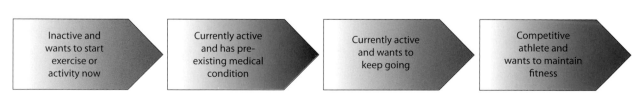

Figure 7.2 General categories of pregnant exerciser

interesting and achievable. Be aware that some women decide to exercise to avoid gaining weight and if an instructor feels that this is the key motivation, the client may require careful management to avoid over-exercising and risking negative effects to the foetus.

Currently active for health

With the growth in awareness and availability of exercise referral schemes, it is the case that many people are becoming regularly active in order to prevent or reduce the effects of medical conditions such as heart disease, diabetes, obesity, arthritis or asthma. This is also generally the case with pregnant women who are concerned that having to reduce their levels of activity during pregnancy may have an adverse effect on their pre-existing medical condition. While during pregnancy it is obvious that the health of the foetus is the main priority, maintaining activity at an appropriate level is unlikely to compromise this and regular exercise should therefore be continued, provided the client is happy with this and appropriate medical advice is sought if necessary.

Currently active

Those women who are already regular exercisers are likely to continue with activity during their pregnancy and although the majority will naturally reduce the intensity and volume of training as the pregnancy progresses, others may try to continue at or even increase pre-pregnancy levels. This is not recommended and an instructor has a duty of care to ensure that any pregnant client with whom they are working is training at an appropriate level to minimise the risk of potential problems with the pregnancy.

Active athlete

Athletes, whether competitive or recreational, are often more aware of their physical limits than non-athletes. When this is the case, during pregnancy mothers-to-be should be encouraged to listen to their bodies and continue to exercise or train within appropriate guidelines and with constant supervision. However, it should be stressed that pregnancy is not the time to try to improve fitness, as it is more appropriate to maintain a reasonable level of fitness in order to make a return to the sport or activity more efficient.

GOAL SETTING

8

KEY POINTS

- Goal setting is the term used when particular information is used in structuring a training plan or exercise programme.
- Regardless of the ability level, fitness status, experience or motivation of the participant, goals should always be agreed by the instructor and the client undertaking the exercise programme.
- Goals are typically divided into two classifications: 'process goals' and 'outcome goals'.
- Form, technique or simply participation in activity are classed as typical process goals.
- Outcome goals are results-related such as in the case of winning or losing.
- Goals tend to be set for particular time periods for example, short term, medium term and long term.
- The acronym SMART or SMARTER, which has been adapted from coaching, is widely used as a common guide to goal setting.
- In most cases it is not appropriate to use weight loss as a process goal.

CONSIDERATIONS FOR GOAL SETTING

Although not used particularly often, or sometimes as well as it should be, goal setting is a relatively simple technique which can provide important information to help an instructor to design and structure a training plan or exercise programme. Goal setting also provides a plan of action that can help the participant to focus on changing particular behaviours. Regardless of the ability level, fitness status, experience or motivation of the participant, goals should be agreed by the instructor and the client as a negotiation. Generally speaking and in relation to physical activity, goals can be split into two types: 'process goals' and 'outcome goals' as shown in table 8.1.

PROCESS GOALS

A process goal is the term that is used where an agreed outcome is broken down into manageable units for the instructor and client to focus on. For example form, technique or simply participation in any activity are classed as process goals as they are related more to the taking part in the activity rather than to the actual results that are achieved.

OUTCOME GOALS

This type of goal is when the instructor or client is concerned only with the ultimate outcome, for example success or failure, winning or losing. In other words, outcome goals are results-related as opposed to process goals which are task-related. During any term of pregnancy, outcome goals are usually not appropriate as they may cause the mother-to-be to focus on unrealistic or unhealthy ideals rather than having the safety of the foetus as the main priority.

TIME PERIOD-RELATED GOALS

Goals can also be set for particular time periods for example, short term, medium term and long term. Even though medium- (trimesters) and long-term (beyond delivery) goals are all appropriate, setting short-term process goals can act as a motivational tool for the mother-to-be to help her maintain appropriate activity throughout pregnancy and into the postnatal period. When agreeing goals with the individual whether short, medium or long term, the acronym SMART or SMARTER is a common guide to goal setting, which includes several common characteristics that are often associated with effective goal setting. While this is normally applied to outcome goals, it can be adapted for process goals during pregnancy. Table 8.2 gives an example of this.

It is important to remember that weight gain in any stage of pregnancy may be affected by a range of factors (see page 25), some of them controllable and some not. It may not therefore be appropriate to use weight as a process goal, however flexible the goal may be, as it can often cause too strong a focus on weight and lead to problems with eating or feelings of anxiety if enough weight is lost, which may occur in women who experience severe nausea or sickness in the first trimester. A focus on well-being or functional ability may be a more suitable and realistic goal and will usually help prevent the development of a potentially obsessive attitude to weight gain during the pregnancy.

Table 8.1 Examples of process and outcome goals	
Process goals	**Outcome goals**
Be able to continue working or exercising throughout pregnancy	Increase my fitness
Keep weight gain within recommended levels	Get back in my pre-pregnancy clothes within six months
Be able to attend antenatal exercise sessions every week	Reduce a dress size
Maintain good posture	

Table 8.2	Examples of SMARTER goals adapted from NCF (1998) – Analysing Your Coaching		
		Outcome goals	**Pregnancy process goals**
	Sample goal	The goal is to lose 0.5kg a week for 10 weeks.	This would be to keep weight gain close to the recommended guidelines of 3lbs/1kg in the 1st trimester.
S	Goals must be: Specific	If the goal of an individual is to lose weight, the amount of weight that is set as the target must be specific. For instance, 0.5kg per week is a specific target.	This is specific as it aims to keep weight gain close to the specific amount of 3lbs/1kg.
M	Targets should be: Measurable	In the example above, 0.5kg is a measurable amount as opposed to 'lose a bit of weight' each week, which could be any amount such as 1g up to 10kg.	3lbs/1kg is a measurable target, provided the starting weight is known.
A	Goals should be: Adjustable	If an individual finds the target too easy or too hard then the coach must adapt the programme to suit, in other words the programme must be adjustable.	During pregnancy there are usually physical changes or issues that affect the amount of weight gained so setting a target of a fixed amount may be inappropriate.
R	Goals must be: Realistic	Set targets that are achievable. 0.5kg weight loss per week is achievable for most people. A target of over 3kg per week might not be achievable or healthy.	Due to sickness or hunger there may be more or less weight gain so having a slightly flexible target may be more realistic at this time.
T	Targets should be: Time based	0.5kg weight loss per week is a short-term target that can lead to an overall loss of about 26kg a year, which may be the long-term goal.	The first trimester lasts from week 1 to week 13 so the time frame is fixed.
E	Goals should be: Exciting	The chances of adherence to the exercise programme are much greater if the programme excites the individual. Looking healthy may excite them more than getting fit.	Keeping to a healthy weight gain is likely to be important to the woman.
R	Goals should be: Recorded	Keeping a written or photographic record of ongoing progress provides a visual stimulus for the individual and can help to continue to motivate them.	Most women have a pregnancy diary which can be used to record weight gain.

Aim	Process goal
I want to get back in pre-pregnancy clothes as soon as possible after my pregnancy.	
I want to keep exercising throughout my pregnancy.	
I do not want to get too round shouldered as a result of the pregnancy.	
I want to keep running at my current pace throughout pregnancy.	

QUALITIES OF
AN INSTRUCTOR

9

KEY POINTS

- Instructing qualities can be broken down into many categories, such as listening skills, motivational skills, delivery skills, observational skills, communication skills and understanding of feedback.
- There are essentially two types of listening which are known as passive and active listening.
- Feedback can come from external sources, which is otherwise known as 'extrinsic feedback' or from internal sources which is known as 'intrinsic feedback'.
- An effective communicator often has good listening, verbal and non-verbal skills (observational).
- It is well known that over 70 per cent of all communication is non-verbal.
- One of the categories of motivation is related to external sources and is known as 'extrinsic motivation' and the other category is related to internal sources and is known as 'intrinsic motivation'.
- Intrinsic motivation is usually linked to the feelings or perceptions of the individual client and is driven by an interest or enjoyment in the task itself.
- External motivation comes from outside the individual and can come from many sources such as extrinsic rewards like money and prizes or in the form of praise from the instructor or family and friends.
- One of the most commonly used methods when delivering exercise sessions is the IDEA method (Introduce, Demonstrate, Execute, Adjust).

RANGE OF QUALITIES

When prescribing and delivering exercise programmes there are many qualities which an instructor should ideally possess that are important, or even vital, when communicating with their clients. Figure 9.1 shows a range of qualities of an instructor that are important for all exercise populations, and in particular for pregnant clients.

LISTENING SKILLS

One of the many common scenarios in instructing is that we often 'hear' but we don't 'listen'. A simple example of this is when we meet someone for the first time and within a few minutes can't remember their name. One of the psychological explanations for this is that we often place more importance on what we have to say than we do on

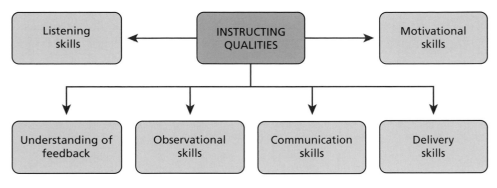

Figure 9.1 Qualities of an instructor

what others have to say and as a result don't try to take in what is said to us. However, the rapport between instructor and mother-to-be is vitally important so 'listening' as a skill becomes one of the main attributes needed by the instructor. Although a complex subject, there are essentially two types of listening which are known as 'passive' and 'active' listening.

Passive listening

An example of passive listening is when we listen to what others have to say without giving any kind of response or acknowledgement. Passive listening however is acceptable in certain situations such as watching a movie, listening to music or when at a theatre because the person speaking does not need to check the understanding of the audience. However, in an instructing situation both the instructor and the client need to know if what has been said has been understood by both parties.

Active listening

This type of listening is evident in a situation where a person listens to a speaker and responds in some way to show whether they understand

the speaker or not as the case may be. In active listening, the instructor generally has to respond to either general statements or specific questions from the client depending on the context or the situation they might be in. For example, scenario 1 overleaf shows an example of a client making a typical statement and how the instructor might deal with this, whereas scenario 2 gives an example of a client asking a typical question and the possible response from the instructor.

As seen from both scenarios, responding to a client's statement or question is not always as straightforward as it might seem. Instructors are often placed in a situation where they have to interpret the information given by a client as there is typically an underlying message that the client is trying to communicate. Every possible scenario can have many outcomes depending on each response from both the client and the instructor. For this reason, experience often proves to be one of the most valuable tools for an instructor, but this obviously takes many years to acquire. Therefore there are several 'top tips' for listening as can be seen in table 9.1 that might help the instructor to improve their listening skills.

Possible scenarios

Scenario 1 – Client statement: 'I think I ran well today.'

This statement requires a response by the instructor to show understanding but the instructor must consider their response carefully. For instance, the client may not have run according to the requirement of the programme so the instructor may need to make the client aware of this. In this scenario the instructor could ask another questions such as 'Did you think that you were running at the correct heart rate level?' or 'Do you think you should be increasing the intensity at this stage in the programme?' This would show that the instructor listened and would open up a debate to help them point out areas for improvement. If the client did run well according to the planned programme, in most cases they would still need encouragement. In this scenario the instructor could say 'You did run well today but tell me, is there anything we might need to adjust in terms of intensity or duration for next time?' Again, this shows understanding but challenges the client to keep thinking about the programme and have a certain degree of responsibility for their own benefit.

Scenario 2 – Client question: 'Do you think I should increase the duration of my run today?'

Again this seems like a fairly harmless question but clients often ask this because they need reinforcement and encouragement as they are not confident enough to take responsibility or ownership of their own programme. One of the ways that an instructor could respond is by saying to the client 'As long as you feel that you are ready, give it a try, but stop if you feel it is too much.' In this way the instructor is showing understanding of the question but reinforcing that it is still the client who has a degree of responsibility for their own programme.

Table 9.1	Top tips for listening

1 As an instructor you need to understand and accept that listening is important.

2 Listen and don't just hear; focus on the speaker and concentrate on what they are saying.

3 Look for the underlying meaning or hidden messages. As in scenarios 1 and 2, is there a hidden message?

4 As an instructor, try not to interrupt the speaker as you may miss important information.

5 Think before responding. It is always best not to respond emotionally. Reflect for a few seconds if you need to.

UNDERSTANDING FEEDBACK

All that the term 'feedback' really means is trying to gather as much information as possible to help the understanding of a particular situation. This can be from the perspective of the instructor getting feedback so that they can check the client's understanding of directions or to help them to improve the skills they are trying to learn. It can also be from the perspective of the client in order to check their own understanding. There are many different sources that instructors and clients can use to gather feedback.

Instructor feedback

It is always important that the instructor receives feedback from the client as often as possible because with pregnant women, health or comfort can change substantially on a daily basis. All exercise programmes therefore, must be as flexible as possible so that the instructor can respond quickly to the client's feedback and accommodate any changes. The instructor will usually receive either verbal or visual feedback directly from the client. Table 9.2 shows typical sources of both verbal and visual feedback from a client.

Client feedback

Feedback that the client receives is generally related to motivational factors or to information regarding the adherence to the exercise programme and meeting specific targets or goals. In terms of the type of client feedback that is available, the information gathered can either come from external sources, which is otherwise known as 'extrinsic feedback' or from internal sources which is known as 'intrinsic feedback'. Table 9.3 gives some examples of both extrinsic and intrinsic feedback sources.

Table 9.2	**Types and examples of instructor feedback sources**
Verbal	**Visual**
Answers: Simple answers to questions such as 'How do you feel on an RPE scale?' will help the instructor to judge the approximate level of intensity that the client is working at.	Technique: By watching the client perform a particular exercise this will help the instructor to check correct execution. Posture and technique are crucial for this population.
Poor response: If the client is unable to communicate with the instructor due to breathlessness, this will give an indication of intensity level.	Discomfort: The instructor should be able to use cues such as facial expressions to judge if the client is coping with a particular exercise level.
Understanding: Correct answers to direct and specific questions will indicate the understanding of particular directions. For example, ask the client to repeat the order of exercise components in their programme to check if they get the correct order.	Sweating: The instructor should always check for indications of overheating for this population. Excessive sweating and redness of the face is one particular sign to look for.

Table 9.3	Types and examples of client feedback sources
Extrinsic	**Intrinsic**
Instructor: There should be directions and guidance from someone qualified to deliver a programme of exercise.	Visual: The use of mirrors to check posture and technique can be a valuable tool when clients first start out.
Peers: Group exercise with other pre-/postnatal women can often result in relevant knowledge being passed on.	Balance: The client's own balance systems in the body will provide information to the brain and this should improve as a result of exercise.
Family/friends: General guidance and support from friends or family can be of great help as clients often have particular people that they will listen to and accept feedback from.	Feel: Client's should be encouraged to stop an exercise if they feel it is uncomfortable or just doesn't 'feel right' and seek guidance from the instructor. Checking technique and posture in a mirror is useful to help the client feel what the body is like during correct execution of an exercise.

Extrinsic feedback

There are many different sources of extrinsic feedback as are described in table 9.3. The term 'extrinsic' simply refers to the client receiving information about the skill or exercise being practised from various external sources such as their instructor or from their fellow peers. For example, an instructor could give feedback by making a comment to the client about their foot, knee, hip and lower back placement during a squat exercise.

Be aware though, that there are often many confusing comments given to clients depending on the exercise environment that they are in. These comments quite often tend to come from overenthusiastic instructors who are not qualified or experienced with this particular population. It is important therefore that qualified instructors should always encourage clients to decline technical advice from non-qualified sources if they feel that the advice is in contradiction to that already given.

Intrinsic feedback

The term 'intrinsic feedback' on the other hand is related to the feelings and senses (relating to their own body) that the client experiences during the performance of a particular exercise. An example of this could be when someone is undertaking a cardiovascular training session during a particular trimester stage and they have the feeling or perception that they are too warm even though the session had been programmed for longer at that particular training intensity. The client should always be encouraged to take note and respond to how they feel as (especially regarding this example of overheating) there are many physiological dangers for this population and exercise should always be stopped if there are any concerns regardless of the programme.

COMMUNICATION SKILLS

In any situation, the term 'communication' is simply a way of getting information across to another person in a way that they can understand. An adept communicator will use a range of skills to ensure that they are clearly understood by others, and that they understand what others are saying (or not saying!). This range includes listening, verbal and non-verbal skills (observational), which combine to make our communication more effective.

Quite often, when certain aspects of communication are missed, the intended message may be misunderstood. Take the example of email or text communications; it is very easy to interpret these in the wrong way as there are no clues to the emotion or the body language of the sender on the screen.

In terms of exercise instruction there are three main methods of communication that are available to the instructor; that of verbal (through the use of the words), para-verbal (through the voice tone and stress on words) and non-verbal (by the use of gestures). It is generally thought that non-verbal communication accounts for around 55 per cent of what others understand, while verbal and para-verbal account for only 7 per cent and 38 per cent respectively. In other words, face-to-face actions are an extremely effective communication tool for the instructor.

Verbal communication

To communicate verbally simply means through the spoken word. Unfortunately, it is a generally accepted fact that humans are not particularly good at retaining much verbal information. This is particularly true of pregnant women who are often very preoccupied and find it hard to concentrate on non-baby related matters (the so called 'baby brain'). In this situation it is wise to limit the amount of verbal information that is given

during instructing otherwise information overload can occur. One of the reasons why this can happen (in very simple terms) is that as human beings we are limited in the amount of information we can take in at any one time because of the capacity of the short-term memory. Information in the short-term memory is regularly transferred to the long-term memory, but if the short-term memory is overloaded it can affect this transfer. We are, however, generally capable of taking in more visual information (through sight) than we are of taking in verbal information. For this

Try this!
You will need pens and paper enough for a few people in a group.

What to do
With a group of people, give each person a pen and paper. Read out a seven-digit number, get them to wait for 5 seconds, then ask them to write down the number (they have to remember it obviously). Do this again but use an eight-digit number and ask them to write it down after a 5 second wait. You should find that most of them would have written the seven-digit number down correctly but completely messed up the eight-digit number.

Why does it happen?
In the field of psychology this is a phenomenon called 'chunking'. Very simply, if the short-term memory thinks it will be overloaded because it is receiving lots of information, it will tend only to remember the first and last bits of the information.

reason it is important that the instructor does not give too much verbal information, particularly during induction sessions, and gives good quality demonstrations.

Para-verbal communication

This particular type of communication relates to the way we use words and how we structure spoken sentences. Placing the stress on different words can change the meaning or emphasis of what we are trying to say, so it is important to ensure that we say what we mean, and in a way that is easily understood.

How we feel as individuals is also reflected in para-verbal communication. For example if we are fed up or excited it comes across in our voice tone so it is important to make sure that as an instructor you sound interested as well as using the right words and positive body language.

Non-verbal communication

To communicate non-verbally is being able to get a particular point (or information) across without speaking. It is well known that over 70 per cent of all communication is non-verbal, which highlights the fact that we often use this method without even thinking. For example, people are often successful in asking for and understanding directions in a non-English speaking country or asking for the bill across a crowded and noisy restaurant. These are just two examples of how effective non-verbal communication can be. There are several types of non-verbal communication (also called 'body language') used when instructing as explained in table 9.4.

Figure 9.2 shows how some of the steps in communication are linked and how it may not be as simple as 'you speak, I understand'. For example, what we are really thinking or wanting to say may not be reflected in the words we use (verbal) but is likely to come across in our body language or tone of voice (para-verbal and non-verbal). Similarly, the listener may 'hear' only the words (verbal) and ignore or miss the accompanying body language that indicates the true meaning of the message (non-verbal). Although both parties have 'listened', there may be a lack of understanding of the underlying message.

Try this!

Say the following phrase out loud placing the emphasis on the word in italics. Note what you feel is the key message that comes across with each phrase.

I said you were probably right

I *said* you were probably right

I said *you* were probably right

I said you were *probably* right

Table 9.4	Categories of non-verbal communication
Category	**Description**
Role model	The way in which you look and dress can often be an influential factor. If you do not look after yourself physically it will give an indication to the client that you are not bothered about fitness.
Body position	The way you position yourself with clients is very important. Don't get too close (in their personal space) as it could intimidate them. Also, do not make contact with the client unless you ask permission first and explain what you are going to do.
Body movements	Simple gestures with the eyes, hands, head, etc., can be very effective. For example, mirroring a particular exercise can often help you to dictate the pace of that exercise.

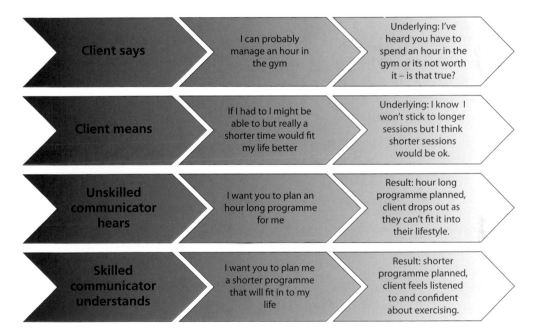

Figure 9.2 Example of a communication link model

It goes without saying that the ability to communicate is crucial and that the more we do it the more we should improve. Many instructors have developed their communication skills over the years by engaging with many clients in many different situations. For those new to working with clients, the 'top tips' for communication in table 9.5 might help you develop your own skills as an instructor.

Table 9.5 Top tips for communication

1 Try to use a range of body language techniques to see if they work.

2 When communicating verbally, pitch the information at the level of the client. Keep it simple!

3 Present yourself as a role model.

4 Ask other instructors to give you feedback on your own communication skills.

MOTIVATIONAL SKILLS

The word 'motivate' is derived from the Latin for 'move' and there are many definitions of the term 'motivation' including 'the driving force by which to achieve specific goals' (in this case they would be exercise-related goals) and 'the internal mechanisms and external stimuli which arouse and direct our behaviour'. In other words, motivation is something that prompts a person to act.

There are several ways in which to motivate people in relation to exercise and activity participation and adherence, but the methods can be grouped into two main categories. One of the categories of motivation is related to external sources and is known more formally as 'extrinsic motivation' while the other category is related to internal sources and is known as 'intrinsic motivation'. It should be remembered however that with this particular population the health of the baby is of paramount importance and any motivational factor, regardless of the type, should have the health of the baby as the main priority. *Note*: Research (in particular by social psychologists) in the area of motivation is vast, therefore it is recommended that the reader refer to other sources if this is an area of interest.

Extrinsic motivation

Within this category, external motivation comes from outside the individual and can come from many sources such as extrinsic rewards like money and prizes, or in the form of praise from the instructor or family and friends. It should be mentioned, however, that it is thought that a focus on extrinsic rewards can lead to a subsequent reduction in internal motivation.

Many people value the comments of instructors and constantly look for praise at every opportunity in order to reinforce that they are doing well in their particular programme and are giving themselves the best opportunity to achieve their goals. Praise is a great motivational tool and can be used in many situations, such as in conjunction with trying to give corrective feedback. However, as an instructor you will often have to correct actions or mistakes and praise can help you to deliver this criticism. This method is called the 'criticism sandwich', as in figure 9.3, and is a good way in which to deliver any corrections or criticism that you might want to make.

For example, an instructor might need to stop a client from pushing themselves too hard during exercise. In this situation they would start with

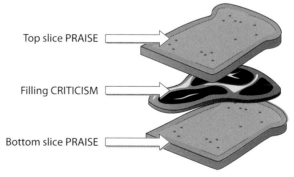

Top slice PRAISE

Filling CRITICISM

Bottom slice PRAISE

Figure 9.3 The 'criticism' sandwich

the top slice of the sandwich by saying something like 'Your running style is excellent'. They would then introduce the filling of the sandwich by adding something like 'You do need to reduce the heart rate to the level we agreed,' and then they would include the bottom slice of the sandwich by adding something like 'This will be great for your baby in the long term'. In other words, the filling of the sandwich is the criticism and the slices of the sandwich just try to make it positive.

Intrinsic motivation

As opposed to extrinsic sources of motivation, intrinsic motivation is usually linked to the feelings or perceptions of the individual client and is driven by an interest or enjoyment in the task itself (in this case the exercise or activity). In relation to this particular population, having fun, feeling competent and a desire to achieve the specific goals are all classed as internal motivational factors. Psychological research often shows that people who tend to be internally motivated are often driven by the need to succeed (known as achievement motivation) and to win, as they usually associate winning with success and losing with failure. For this population, however, it is up to the instructor to impress upon the client that success is by way of achieving the goals that have been agreed by the instructor and the client. It can sometimes be the case that someone who is internally driven who does not experience at least a small amount of success is likely to blame themselves for the 'failure', thinking that they do not have the ability to be successful. Unfortunately there are only a small percentage of people who would use failure as the motivation to try again because they thought that their failure was due to lack of effort, therefore, it is for this reason that

Table 9.6	Top tips for motivating
1	Use the criticism sandwich when trying to correct (praise – criticism – praise).
2	Give lots of praise to beginners to activities to help them develop.
3	Try to be positive at all times to create an atmosphere to build self-esteem.
4	Only give praise when the clients deserve it.
5	Stress the importance of participation and taking part and not just achieving goals.
6	Try to set achievable targets so that clients can experience some level of success.

short-term goals should be made achievable and regularly adapted to suit the programme.

It is recommended that instructors try to be as positive as they can at all times as this kind of environment will help build client self-esteem and confidence whereas a negative attitude will only create a fear of failure and lack of self-esteem. That doesn't mean that instructors should always praise and compliment as corrections can always be given in a positive manner. As with all instructor qualities, experience is invaluable – however, the 'top tips' in table 9.6 should help instructors with regards to motivating their clients.

DELIVERY SKILLS

As an instructor delivering exercise programmes to this particular population, it is important that the methods of delivery are as good and safe as they possibly can be. There are many methods of delivery that can be used and most instructors will have their own preference as to which suits a particular situation.

The IDEA method of delivery

One of the most commonly used methods when delivering exercise sessions (in all situations and not just with pregnant women) is the IDEA method as shown in figure 9.4.

Introduce

This might sound straightforward, but instructors often forget to introduce the exercise that they are about to demonstrate. For example, 'This is the chest press which is going to help build strength in the chest and back of the arms' is all that is required to set the scene for the client for that particular exercise.

Demonstrate

As was explained in relation to information overload, try to limit the amount of verbal information and rely more on visual demonstrations. Having said that, it is crucial that the instructor is able to demonstrate the technique of the exercise correctly so that the client can copy what is done. If the instructor is not able to demonstrate for some reason, then they will have no other choice than to talk the client through the exercise. The instructor should also demonstrate the exercise at the speed at which they intend the client to perform the same exercise. Once the client is doing the exercise the instructor can use a mirror technique to reinforce the speed of execution.

Execute

This is just another term for carrying out the chosen exercise. Once the instructor has demonstrated the chosen exercise, the client should then be given the opportunity to try it.

Adjust

This is just another term for correcting errors by giving feedback as covered earlier in this chapter. If the client accurately follows the demonstration of the instructor then there should be little to adjust. The instructor might want to correct things such as posture and speed of the exercise at this point.

It is advisable to always try to improve on delivery as an instructor. One of the ways to do this is to first assess the delivery of current performance in order to identify any areas that could be improved upon. There are many ways in which to do this such as by using a self-assessment score sheet (see table 9.7) in which instructors rate their own performance in different areas relating to delivery in a practical situation. A self-assessment sheet is normally completed at the end of the delivery of a session so that the details are still fresh in the mind of the instructor in order for an accurate recall to be made.

The self-assessment score sheet is designed such that the more the instructor is in agreement

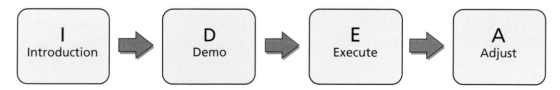

Figure 9.4 The IDEA method of delivery

Table 9.7	Instructor self-assessment sheet				

Give yourself a score for each statement. 1 = totally disagree and 5 = totally agree

	1	2	3	4	5
My instructions are always brief and straight to the point.					
I always demonstrate correctly.					
I tend to give demonstrations from different angles so that the client can see.					
I never over-complicate instructions.					
When giving feedback to clients it is mostly positive.					
Most feedback I give is information about the exercise and not judging the client.					
I am usually quite consistent in the way I give feedback.					
I try to listen to what clients have to say as much as possible.					
I always try to encourage participation as well as achievement of goals.					
Total score =					

with the statement the higher the score should be (scoring between 1 and 5). When the instructor has given a score to each statement, they should add up all the scores to give a total. Generally speaking, the higher the overall score the 'better' the delivery should be. If the score is more than 27 points overall then it is suggesting that the instructor must be delivering reasonably well. If however the score is less than 27 points then maybe the instructor should reflect on the way they deliver in order to try to improve, particularly in relation to the statements which scored the lowest. For instance, if an instructor feels that they are giving too many instruction points during an exercise session they should try to use non-verbal communication every time they feel they need to point something out. For example, if they feel that they need to emphasise breathing technique, then they should demonstrate so that the client can see them and will be able to copy them.

INSTRUCTING // STYLES

10

KEY POINTS

- There are many recognised instructing styles such as autocratic, democratic, command and reciprocal.
- The autocratic instructing style is generally split into two distinct types, one type known as 'telling' and the other type known as 'selling'.
- The democratic instructing style is split into two distinct types known as 'sharing' and 'allowing'.
- The command instructing style is one in which there is direct instruction and the instructor makes all the decisions for the clients to follow.
- The reciprocal style is one in which the client takes some responsibility (with instructor guidance) for their own development throughout their programme of exercise.
- Regardless of the style of instruction used, it is important for the instructor to have a plan of what they are doing and any eventuality that may occur.
- Instructors often employ more than one method of instructing during the same session.
- Many people new to instructing tend to adopt the command style because they themselves were exposed to it or because they are able to avoid questions by just dictating the process due to a lack of in-depth knowledge.

INSTRUCTING STYLES

There are many different ways in which people instruct (known as an 'instructing style') and in some cases more than one method is employed during the same session. Although this differs depending on the individual taking part in the session, with this particular population, the way someone instructs can be vitally important not just for safety reasons but for the purpose of achieving agreed targets.

Perhaps the two most commonly recognised instructing styles that have been developed primarily from a coaching background are those known as 'autocratic' (do as I say) and 'democratic' (clients help in decision making).

AUTOCRATIC AND DEMOCRATIC INSTRUCTION STYLES

The autocratic instructing style is generally split into two distinct types or subcategories. One type is known as 'telling' and the other type is known as 'selling'. The democratic instruction style is also split into two distinct types known as 'sharing' and 'allowing'. Table 10.1 describes the subcategories of autocratic and democratic types of instruction. As mentioned before, instructors do not usually use one style of instructing throughout a session but often use a variety of styles or types depending on the particular situation at the time. There are however other instructing styles that are useful for this particular population in an exercise environment.

For example, other styles that have been identified are those such as 'command' and 'reciprocal' style.

COMMAND INSTRUCTING STYLE

This particular style is one in which there is direct instruction and the instructor makes all the decisions for the clients to follow. This style of instructing normally assumes that the instructor is well qualified and experienced in this area and knows what they are talking about, therefore the client listens. This type of instruction is often employed by elite-level coaches.

Many people new to instructing tend to adopt the command style for various reasons. One reason is often that it was the style they themselves were

Table 10.1 Autocratic and democratic instructing styles and their types			
Autocratic		**Democratic**	
Telling	Selling	Sharing	Allowing
Instructor decides on what is to be done	Instructor decides what is to be done	Instructor outlines session to the clients	Instructor outlines the session to the clients
Clients not involved in any decisions	Instructor explains objectives	Instructor invites ideas from the clients	Instructor defines conditions
Instructor defines what and how to do it	Clients encouraged to question and confirm understanding	Instructor makes decisions based on clients' suggestions	Clients explore possible ideas.
Clients told the exercises	Instructor defines what and how to do it	Instructor defines what and how to do it	Clients make the decision
	Instructor explains the object of the session and purpose of each exercise	Instructor identifies a session outline	Clients define what and how to do it
	Clients ask questions	Clients identify possible exercises for the session	Instructor identifies a session
		Instructor selects from the suggestions	Instructor defines conditions of the session
			Clients identify exercises for the session that meet the instructor's conditions

81

exposed to, or because they are able to avoid questions by just dictating the process which shows a lack of in-depth knowledge. However, for those that are suitably qualified and knowledgeable the command style can often be a useful method for those clients who do not feel confident enough to take ownership of their own programme.

RECIPROCAL INSTRUCTING STYLE (ALSO KNOWN AS COOPERATIVE STYLE)

This particular style is one in which the client takes some responsibility for their own development throughout their programme of exercise (although this is monitored and guided by the instructor).

The reciprocal style still allows the instructor to ultimately make the decisions (as in the command style), but it feels as though the clients have had a say in the decision-making process.

Regardless of what style of instructing is used, it is important for the instructor to have a plan of what they are doing and any eventuality that may occur. Planning is essential to the success of any exercise programme.

PLANNING

KEY POINTS

- One reason that planning of a particular programme of exercise is vital is so that the short-, medium- and long-term goals can potentially be achieved.
- A typical exercise planning pathway follows the stages of: goal setting, identify fitness components, test fitness components, periodising a programme and regular testing.
- A typical exercise planning pathway for a pregnant woman follows the stages of: goal setting, identify fitness history, periodising a programme for trimesters one, two and three and the postnatal period, monitoring and feedback.
- Goals should have the benefit of the health of the baby as the main priority as opposed to any unrealistic goals for the underlying purpose of the mother-to-be's vanity.
- Fitness components should always be identified that are specific to the agreed goals so that the design of the exercise programme will be specific to the individual and their needs.
- The fitness history of the client should always be established prior to the undertaking of any programme of exercise.
- The periodised training programme should always be flexible as it is dependent on many variables that occur during pregnancy.
- Fitness levels are likely to fall towards the end of the pregnancy so the use of standard fitness testing will be inappropriate at this time.

THE IMPORTANCE OF PLANNING

There are many good reasons why planning should be done for each new client yet there are too many incidences of instructors not using carefully prepared exercised programmes when working with particular clients over a period of time. For example, if a client's goals have been identified and agreed, then planning of a particular programme of exercise is vital so that the short-, medium- and long-term goals can be achieved, providing the correct fitness components have been identified and targeted. There are a number of programming models available, however many exercise programmes often follow the path identified in figure 11.1.

Note: It is assumed that clients have been fully screened prior to any stage of planning taking place.

GOAL SETTING

The planning pathway has been designed with simplicity in mind. Before trying to identify any specific exercises, the goals of the client should always be discussed. It is important to remember at this stage that all goals should have the benefit of the health of the baby as the main priority as opposed to any unrealistic goals for the underlying purpose of vanity of the mother-to-be.

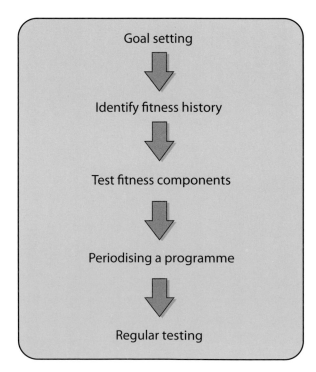

Figure 11.1 Typical exercise planning pathway

IDENTIFY FITNESS COMPONENTS

Once the goals of the client have been identified and agreed with the instructor, then the fitness components (see chapter 12) that are specific to the agreed goals need to be identified. For example, if the mother-to-be wishes to be able to carry her child without any excessive muscular strain and resultant postural problems, then improvement in upper body strength would be identified as a required component of fitness and exercises should be given that promote upper body strength in a lifting-type motion.

TEST FITNESS COMPONENTS

Each of the identified fitness components should be tested so that it provides baseline data of the current level of the client. This data can then be used for comparison purposes when further testing is carried out at later stages. It should be stressed however, that only submaximal testing should be done with this population (see *Practical Fitness Testing* by Morc Coulson (A&C Black) for further information on testing).

PERIODISING A PROGRAMME

The fitness components that are identified must be put into a comprehensive programme as it is important that some components are developed first before others can be. For instance, having good arm strength is not much use without strong core stabilisers to support the spine during lifting. This overall planning is better known as periodisation. Periodisation is often described as the systematic planning of a training programme and the manipulation of the training variables (frequency, intensity, time and type) for a specific time period (cycles or phases as they are known). Microcycles, mesocycles and macrocycles are the common cycles or periods associated with periodisation, but for this population it is probably better to use the trimesters as definite training periods unless working with a client who is only contemplating pregnancy.

As with all training programmes a periodised training programme should be flexible as it is dependent on many variables such as adaptation of the individual, success of the programme and injury.

REGULAR TESTING

Finally, each identified component of fitness that was tested at the start of the programme should be tested at regular intervals in order to assess the effectiveness of the programme. However, with a pregnant client fitness levels are likely to fall towards the end of the pregnancy so the use of standard fitness testing will be inappropriate at this time. Instead, focus on attendance or how they are feeling as a way of monitoring the programme. Figure 11.2 shows a suggested exercise planning pathway for a pregnant client.

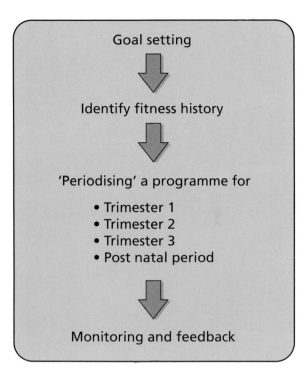

Figure 11.2 Suggested pregnancy planning pathway

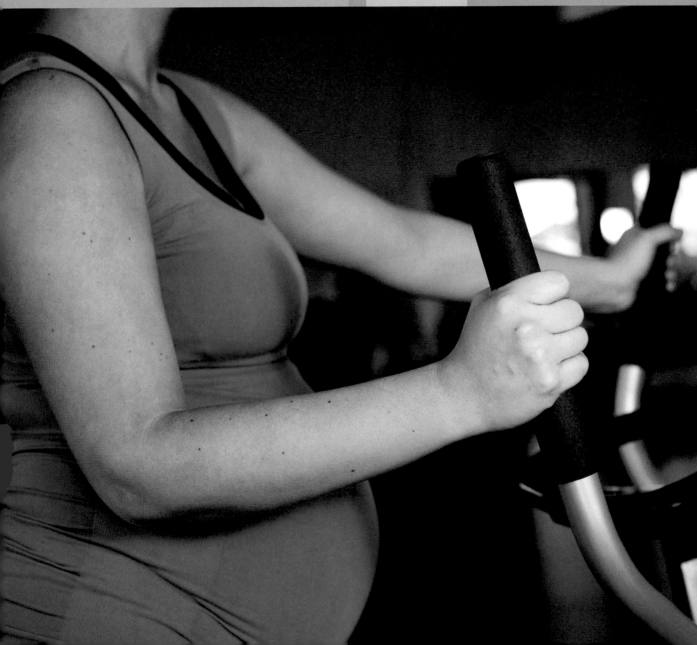

PART **THREE**

PRACTICAL APPLICATION

COMPONENTS OF FITNESS

// 12

KEY POINTS

- 'Components of fitness' as they are known, should always be addressed when designing an exercise programme.
- The components of physical fitness covered in this book are cardiovascular endurance, muscular strength and endurance, flexibility and motor skills.
- Volume, intensity and frequency must be taken into consideration regardless of the component of fitness being trained.
- Cardiovascular endurance is the ability of the heart and lungs to deliver oxygen (work aerobically) to the working muscles of the body and for those muscles to use this oxygen in order to do work, and is measured in $mlO_2.kg^{-1}min^{-1}$.
- One method of measuring exercise intensity is to use a scale known as the 'rate of perceived exertion' (RPE).
- Muscular strength can be described as the maximum amount of force a muscle or muscle group can generate. Muscular endurance can be described as the ability of a muscle or muscle group to perform repeated contractions against a resistance over a period of time.
- Flexibility is defined as 'the ability to move a joint through its complete range of motion'. Stretching can be described as 'an exercise done to either maintain or improve flexibility'.
- There are essentially two types of balance: 'static balance' and 'dynamic balance'. Static balance – this simply means to maintain equilibrium (balance) in a stationary position. Dynamic balance – this means to maintain equilibrium (balance) while in motion.
- Proprioceptors are tiny sensors in the body that detect tension in tendons. This information can then be used to work out the position of joints which is then relayed to the brain.

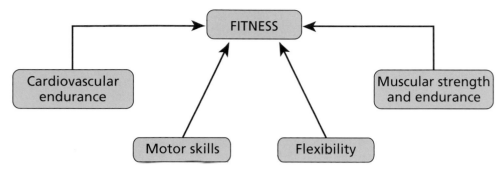

Figure 12.1 Components of fitness

THE IMPORTANCE OF COMPONENTS OF FITNESS

As with any population, there are many areas, or 'components of fitness' as they are known, that instructors should address when designing an exercise programme. These do vary from text to text however, but for the purpose of this book and in relation to pregnancy, the components of fitness that are suggested to be of major importance are those that are shown in figure 12.1. It should also be stressed at this point that each component of fitness should be approached from the point of view that any advice or programming should always be for the benefit of the mother and baby.

Each of the fitness components identified can be addressed in an exercise programme and can be adapted individually without any of the others necessarily improving. Therefore, depending on the type of regular exercise carried out an individual might improve in one or more of the fitness components but not necessarily in all of them.

The components of physical fitness covered in this book are cardiovascular endurance, muscular strength and endurance, flexibility and motor skills (of which there are several subcomponents). See the task in the 'Try this!' box to identify which components of fitness you think are required for the range of different activities listed.

CARDIOVASCULAR ENDURANCE

Quite often you will hear the term 'endurance training' as opposed to the term 'cardiovascular endurance training' even though they really just mean the same thing (or they should do!). You will also hear this referred to as 'aerobic endurance', but whatever the term used it always refers to the ability of the heart and lungs to deliver oxygen (work aerobically) to the working muscles of the body and for those muscles to use this oxygen in order to do work (exercise, sport, events, activities, etc.). It is obvious therefore that oxygen is very important in the process of providing the body with energy to do work.

Cardiovascular endurance is a particular ability that is often measured using various types of fitness tests (such as the multi-stage fitness test or step tests) which all measure (usually indirectly) the amount of oxygen the body is able to deliver to the working muscles. Regardless of the test being done, any test of cardiovascular endurance can result (normally after an equation has been calculated) in a measurement called 'volume of oxygen'

Try this!

For each sport or type of exercise below place a tick in the box or boxes that a component of fitness relates to.

	Cardio	Muscular strength	Muscular endurance	Flexibility	Balance	Speed	Agility	Power
Aerobics								
Aqua								
Ballroom dancing								
Bowling								
Cycling								
Darts								
Gymnastics								
High jump								
Resistance training								
Running								
Swimming								
Tai Chi								
Tennis								
Walking								
Yoga								

(VO_2) with VO_2max being the maximum amount of oxygen that can be delivered to and used by the working muscles. It makes sense therefore that the more oxygen a person can get to their muscles the more exercise they will be able to do.

With regards to pregnancy, a pregnant woman may just want to maintain her cardiovascular fitness level whereas a woman who is planning pregnancy may want to improve her level prior to conception.

Benefits of cardiovascular training

There are many published benefits that are associated with undertaking regular sessions of cardiovascular training that include both physiological and psychological areas. Figure 12.2 shows just some of the many benefits.

Areas for consideration

When trying to prescribe or programme cardiovascular training, there are several areas to consider. Volume, intensity and frequency of the activities must be taken into consideration as they play an important role with respect to maintenance, improvement, overtraining and prevention of injury.

Volume

The term 'volume' is just another name for the amount of exercise or activity done (in this case cardiovascular exercise which is normally measured in mileage or time). Sometimes the individual might not know the distance being covered so they might prefer to measure the training volume by using time. For instance, a training programme that has three 5km runs each week or three 30 minute runs each week.

Intensity

The term 'intensity' simply refers to 'how hard' the exercise or activity is. In other words, in the case of cardiovascular endurance, how hard would it be to cycle or run, etc., at a particular pace? As the intensity of the exercise increases (this can be running faster or cycling uphill, etc.), the amount of oxygen required to cope with the demand of the exercise also increases, therefore the heart rate increases in proportion to get more oxygen around the body. This increase in heart rate due to an increase in exercise intensity is known as a

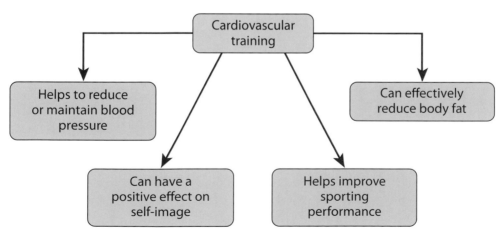

Figure 12.2 Benefits of cardiovascular training

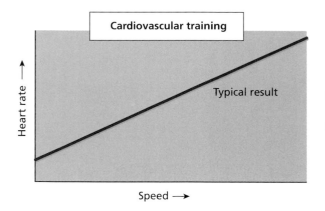

Figure 12.3 Graph showing heart rate against speed

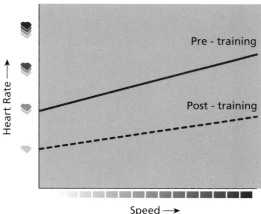

Figure 12.4 Graph showing heart rate against speed for pre- and post-training

'linear relationship'. In other words, if the intensity of the exercise was steadily increased and the heart rate measured after each increase, the points on the graph would be close to a straight line as can be seen in figure 12.3.

This linear relationship between heart rate and intensity is really useful for tracking fitness levels. For instance, if a test is set up to measure the heart rate of an individual after increasing the speed (in a measured way) during a run, it is known as taking a 'baseline' measurement. If the same test is done several weeks later and the measurement line is lower (as in figure 12.4) this shows that the individual is fitter, as the speeds they are training at are maintained with a lower heart rate.

It must be noted however that this type of testing would be better to do in the months leading up to conception as an increase in cardiovascular fitness would not usually be a goal during pregnancy itself.

Frequency

This is a term which simply states 'how often' the exercise or activity takes place. For example, an individual might have three training sessions per week but only do cardiovascular training in two of them, therefore, the frequency of training is three times per week but the frequency of cardiovascular training is two times per week.

Monitoring cardiovascular intensity

There are several methods of prescribing (and actually monitoring) a particular cardiovascular exercise intensity for an individual (how hard the individual should exercise). These methods include heart rate, metabolic equivalents (MET), rating of perceived exertion (RPE), self-perception and communication-based methods such as the 'talk test'. In order to ensure that an individual is exercising at the correct prescribed intensity level within the required training zone one of these methods should be employed (bearing in mind that there are errors associated with each method).

Heart rate

One of the most common methods of prescribing or monitoring cardiovascular intensity is by using the heart rate method. As the intensity of the exercise increases, the heart rate of the individual doing the exercise increases in a linear fashion as is shown in figure 12.3. Generally speaking there are training zones that are related to a percentage of maximum heart rate (see figure 12.5) that have been devised with certain goals in mind. For example, if an individual has a goal of developing aerobic fitness, it would be recommended that they exercise at a heart rate level of between 70 and 80 per cent of their maximum (the aerobic zone). This can be written as 70–80%HRM. If the goal was mainly weight loss then a heart rate level of between 60 and 70 per cent of the individual's maximum would be recommended.

However, the maximum heart rate of the individual must be known in order to calculate a percentage of it. There are two ways in which maximum heart rate can be established, either by testing or by estimation. It is not ethical or safe to test a pregnant woman's maximum heart rate as this requires an all-out maximum effort therefore an estimation known as 'predicted maximum heart rate' must be made. Instructors should remember that if they are using prediction methods such as the Karvonen formula, resting heart rate can increase by up to 15bpm during pregnancy.

Predicted maximum heart rate

There are many different published formulae that can be used to predict maximum heart rate. One of the easiest to remember is the following formula (even though there can be an error of plus or minus 12bpm using this method):

$$\text{Maximum heart rate} = 220 - \text{age}$$

For example, a 23-year-old person would have a predicted maximum heart rate of 197bpm (220 − 23) and a 45-year-old person would have a predicted maximum heart rate of 175bpm (220 − 45). Even though there are errors associated with this method of estimating maximum heart rate, it is a common method that is suitable for the health and fitness industry and in particular for this population as it doesn't take resting heart rate into account.

Once the predicted maximum heart rate is established using the 220 − age formula it is then possible to calculate the percentage of heart rate maximum that is required for training purposes for the individual. Having established the maximum heart rate for the individual, it is then multiplied by the chosen percentage to give the training heart rate maximum in beats per minute.

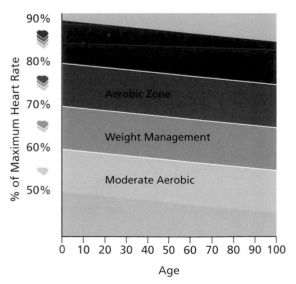

Figure 12.5 General heart rate training zones

Example

Let us assume that it had been agreed between an instructor and a client that the training intensity would be programmed between 70 and 80 per cent of the client's maximum heart rate (this is in the aerobic zone as can be seen in figure 12.5). Let us also make the assumption for this example that the client is 32 years of age. It is the role of the instructor to calculate the individual's training intensity heart rates of between 70 and 80 per cent of maximum as follows:

Step 1:
Predicted maximum heart rate for the individual is 220 − age (32) = 188bpm

Step 2:
70% of maximum (188bpm) = (188/100 × 70) = 131bpm
80% of maximum (188bpm) = (188/100 × 80) = 150bpm
Note: Round the answer to the nearest whole number.

In this example, the 32-year-old wishing to exercise in the aerobic zone (70–80 per cent maximum heart rate) would need to keep their heart rate level between 131bpm and 150bpm.

The steps shown in the example can be used to calculate heart rate for training within a particular prescribed zone. This, however, would be more suited to women who are planning to get pregnant (especially when prescribing exercise in the anaerobic zone).

Table 12.1 shows the age-related heart rate training zones for aerobic type activities that are recommended by the Royal College of Obstetricians and Gynaecologists (RCOG). *Note*: These are guidelines that should be followed by women who are pregnant. It should be stressed however that this is a general guideline for women who have a history of being active prior to conception.

Rate of perceived exertion (RPE)
Another method of setting and monitoring the appropriate exercise intensity for an individual is to use a scale known as the 'rate of perceived exertion' (RPE) scale, as shown in figure 12.6. This scale was first introduced by Dr Gunnar Borg and

Table 12.1	Aerobic heart rate training zones for pregnancy
Maternal age	**Heart rate target zone (beats/min)**
Less than 20 years	140–155
20–29 years	135–150
30–39 years	130–145
Over 40 years	125–140

is the preferred method of monitoring intensity of both the RCOG and the American Congress of Obstetricians and Gynecologists (ACOG), who suggest that the increased resting heart and increased stroke volumes associated with pregnancy make the use of heart rate monitoring a difficult task.

The RPE scale is a method often used by instructors (and frequently by researchers) to obtain the subjective feelings of the individual (how the individual feels) during exercise by asking how they rate their own effort. The estimation of the intensity level on the scale perceived by the individual during cardiovascular exercise has been found to

6–20 scale	0–10 scale	Estimate of %MHR
6	0 Nothing at all	
7 Very, very light	0.3	
8	0.5 Extremely weak	50%
9 Very light	0.7	55%
10	1 Very weak	60%
11 Fairly light	1.5	65%
12	2 Weak	70%
13 Somewhat hard	2.5	75%
14	3 Moderate	80%
15 Hard	4	85%
16	5 Strong	88%
17 Very hard	6	92%
18	7 Very strong	96%
19 Very, very hard	8	98%
20	9	100%
	10 Extremely strong	
	11 Absolute maximum	

Figure 12.6 Borg RPE scales. Adapted from *ACSM Guidelines for Exercise Testing and Prescription* (2006)

correlate highly with heart rate. For example, an effort rating of very hard (which is 17 on the 6–20 scale) would usually correspond to a heart rate of approximately 170bpm. For this reason the RPE scale is widely used as an alternative to heart rate as a method of measuring intensity.

There are two RPE scales that are commonly used: the 6–20 scale and the revised 0–10+ scale known as the category ratio scale (CR-10 scale). When used, an individual is shown the scale during exercise and asked how they feel compared to the words on the scale. This response by the individual is then used to correspond to either the estimate of the percentage of heart rate maximum (as shown in column 3 of figure 12.6) or to the actual heart rate of the individual. For example, if the individual states that they feel as though the exercise is 'somewhat hard', this equates to level 13 on the 6–20 scale which then corresponds to a heart rate of 130bpm or an estimation of about 70 per cent of their MHR.

Depending on the goal of the individual, the instructor can recommend an RPE level for the individual to exercise at without the need to monitor heart rate. It also allows the individual to train on their own and be able to monitor their own intensity quite easily. Even though the psychological subjective perception of exercise intensity correlates well with heart rate, it is important to note that various individuals carrying out exactly the same exercise session might report different levels of RPE. There are many factors that could affect this perception rating such as fitness levels, exercise familiarity and illness.

MUSCULAR STRENGTH AND ENDURANCE

The terms 'muscular strength' and 'muscular endurance' are both considered to be components of fitness that can be trained independently. For example, a person can have good muscular strength but poor muscular endurance, or the other way round. Muscular strength and muscular endurance can both be achieved by way of resistance training which could be in the form of free weights, resistance machines or body weight.

These particular descriptions suggest that muscular strength relates to training with heavy weights and doing few repetitions, whereas muscular endurance would be related to training with lighter weights but doing a higher number of repetitions.

Resistance training is sometimes associated with an increase in muscle size (an increase in cross-sectional area to be precise), which is called 'hypertrophy', although this is not as easy to achieve as some people might think. In order to gain considerable muscle size there are many factors that must be considered. Some of these factors include the genetics of the individual needing to be right (a good proportion of fast-twitch fibres in the muscles), the individual needs to train hard using weights that are appropriate and their nutrition has to be good enough to

What do these terms mean?

- Muscular strength can be described as the maximum amount of force a muscle or muscle group can generate.
- Muscular endurance can be described as the ability of the muscle or muscle group to perform repeated contractions against a resistance over a period of time.

What does this term mean?

Resynthesis is a term that is used to describe what happens when protein in the muscles breaks down then rebuilds again.

support the training and help protein resynthesis within the muscles.

Following a resistance training session (up to two days afterwards), whether the training bias was for muscular strength or endurance, it is common for individuals to experience pain or stiffness within the muscles that have been trained. This sensation of pain or stiffness is termed 'delayed onset of muscle soreness' or DOMS. Even though the mechanism of DOMS is not fully understood, instructors should advise individuals to do some light aerobic exercise (such as brisk walking or cycling) immediately following a resistance training session. There is a great deal of evidence suggesting that this can reduce the effect of DOMS by flushing away the build-up of toxins that is thought to be responsible.

Try this!

Identify a location in the body for each muscle. Write down where you think each muscle attaches and what function it will have in pregnancy.

Rectus abdominus (RA)	Lower ribs to pelvis	Support uterus
Triceps		
Biceps		
Pectorals		
Trapezius		
Latissimus dorsi		
Deltoids		
Quadriceps		
Hamstrings		
Calf		
Tibialis anterior		
Hip abductors		
Hip adductors		
Gluteus maximus		
Hip flexors		
Transversus abdominis (TA)		
Erector spinae		

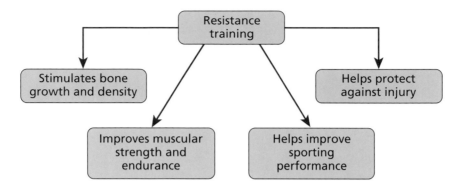

Figure 12.7 Benefits of resistance training

Benefits of resistance training

Like all other components of fitness there are many benefits of resistance training such as those outlined in figure 12.7. Research-based evidence produced over many decades has consistently shown that muscular strain imposed on bone, as a result of resistance training, can help stimulate bone growth which would obviously help to protect against breaks (the amount of strain is still under debate) and improve functional capacity. Another commonly agreed benefit of resistance training is that an increase in muscular strength can help to prevent muscle strains (a strain is the term used to define a tear in the muscle tissue). An increase in muscular strength and endurance therefore would also be a benefit for particular sports or events as these are important components of fitness in almost all physical activities including exercise-related activities such as jogging, cycling and resistance training.

Areas for consideration

As when prescribing cardiovascular training, the individual components of volume, intensity and frequency also have to be considered when prescribing any form of resistance training as these components can also play an important role with respect to improvement in muscular strength/endurance, overtraining, posture and prevention of injury.

Volume

The volume of a particular exercise, in relation to resistance training, can be measured in one of two ways:

- Sets x repetitions or
- Sets x repetitions x load

The term 'load' when used in relation to resistance training simply refers to the amount of weight that is lifted during a particular exercise and the term 'repetitions' refers to the number of times that the load is lifted without a break and before fatigue sets in. The term 'sets' just refers to how many times this is repeated with a break between each set. For example, for an individual who performs three sets of 10 repetitions of 80kg, the volume can be calculated as either 30 reps (at 80kg) or 2400kg.

Intensity

Training intensity (otherwise known as the load) is simply the amount of weight that is to be lifted during a particular exercise as previously discussed. Many published guidelines often refer to 'repetition maximum' or RM. This means the maximum weight that can be lifted for a specific number of repetitions. For example, if a guideline states that the performer should train with 10RM loads, then this is the maximum weight that can be lifted by the performer for 10 repetitions (and they would fail on the 11th repetition).

Intensity can also be expressed as a percentage of the maximum weight that an individual can lift once. You will often see a programme written where the intensity of an exercise might be set at 80 per cent of maximum. This means 80 per cent of the maximum weight that the individual can lift. The problem with this method is that individuals need to be tested in order to find out what their maximum capability would be, which is not recommended either prior to, during or after pregnancy, so multiple repetitions would be advised.

Frequency

This definition is exactly the same as it is for cardiovascular endurance. In this particular case, frequency refers to how many times per week an individual would perform resistance training. Be aware that this refers to the individual muscles being trained and not just the training session. For example, an individual might do three training sessions a week but only train a particular muscle or muscle group (chest, for instance) once therefore the training frequency for the chest is once per week. A better term might therefore be 'muscle group frequency'.

Monitoring resistance intensity (prior to conception only)

When prescribing a particular intensity of a resistance exercise for an individual (how heavy the weight should be), the intensity of the exercise to be performed can be expressed by using a percentage of the maximum capability of that individual. For instance, it has already been stated that the maximum weight that an individual is capable of lifting once is known as 1 repetition maximum (1RM) so it follows that a percentage of this maximum could then be prescribed for the individual depending on their particular goal. For example, if a client wanted to increase her upper-body strength prior to conception the instructor could prescribe appropriate exercises 70 and 80 per cent of 1RM capability.

This method has a disadvantage in that the maximum capability of the individual must be found first before a percentage of this can be calculated. As the individual would have to perform to maximum capability, the risk of injury would be high and not inline with recommended guidelines (see page 56). An easier method would be to use a multiple of the repetition maximum such as 10RM or 15RM. This means the maximum weight the individual can lift 10 or 15 times respectively, as previously explained.

The American College of Sports Medicine (ACSM) guidelines for strength and endurance are also given in multiples of RM. When prescribing resistance exercises for the purpose of gaining muscular strength benefits, weights within the range of 8RM and 12RM are recommended and for muscular endurance benefits weights within the range of 10RM and 15RM apply.

Research shows that the multiple of repetition maximum that is performed by the individual correlates to a percentage of the maximum capability of that individual as shown in table 12.2 which is adapted from *Essentials of Strength Training and Conditioning* by Baechle and Earle (2008).

When trying to establish the amount of weight (load) that an individual can lift for a specific number of repetitions (multiple repetitions maximum) a procedure should be used that ensures that the individual is sufficiently warmed up in order to minimise the risk of injury. If it has been prescribed by the instructor that an intensity of 12RM is going to be used for a particular exercise, then the client should perform several repetitions of a light weight first. After a short rest period, more weight should be added, depending on the ease of the first set, for the client to perform several more repetitions. This process should be repeated until only 12 repetitions and not 13 can be performed at a particular weight, however,

Table 12.2	Multiple of repetition maximum compared to % of maximum
Repetition max (RM)	% of max
1	100
2	93.5
3	91
4	88.5
5	86
6	83.5
7	81
8	78.5
9	76

the instructor should ensure that sufficient rest is given between sets for the client to fully recover. Normally, 1–3 minutes should be enough for full recovery depending on how much energy the client expended. The final weight (or load) that the individual was able to lift 12 times, and not 13, would then be the 12RM weight for that particular exercise. Depending on the resistance training programme that had been prescribed, this process would then be repeated for all resistance exercises that had been chosen.

For progression purposes and assuming that the multiple repetition maximum chosen is to remain constant, when the individual is capable of comfortably performing the chosen RM, the weight can then be increased by a small amount. If the individual cannot perform the number of chosen repetitions at the increased weight they must revert back to the original weight. This type of in-built progression is easy to implement and enables the instructor to empower the individual to take control of their own progression monitoring. However, it may not be appropriate to establish weight limits in this way unless the individual has good technique and is comfortable and familiar with the procedure.

FLEXIBILITY

It is common for the terms 'flexibility' and 'stretching' to be used interchangeably, but this is a mistake as they are very different in practice. Flexibility is defined as 'the ability to move a joint through its complete range of motion'. Stretching however is a term that relates to specific training as is described in the commonly seen definition 'an exercise done to either maintain or improve flexibility'. Thus it can be seen by the definition of flexibility that it is an ability that someone has, whereas stretching is a physical act performed to help or improve that ability.

It should be understood that flexibility is 'joint specific' in that an individual may be flexible in one joint but not necessarily in another. Although over-flexibility (known as 'hyper-flexibility') is linked to possible joint instability and injury, one of the main benefits of maintaining a reasonable range of motion of joints is to allow individuals to carry out daily activities for as long as possible throughout their lives. As some sports require a great amount of flexibility, athletes may be willing to accept the greater risk of joint injury in later life. Reduced flexibility during pregnancy is not normally an issue due to the effects of hormones in the body (see page 16) so instructors should take this into account when prescribing and monitoring flexibility exercises.

Types of stretches

There are many types of stretching exercises that can be used including static, dynamic, PNF and ballistic stretches. Although it is often stated that stretching can help prevent injury, there is little evidence to support this and it is thought that people often stretch because of habit. It has also been shown that a high degree of flexibility (hyper-flexibility) as well as a low degree of flexibility can increase injury risk and cause postural problems.

It is generally recommended that people with tight muscles would probably benefit most from stretching whereas people who are naturally supple should not engage in more than light stretching. As one of the effects of pregnancy is to increase range-of-motion and suppleness it is unlikely that stretching exercises would be a focus of any prescribed programme. It is useful however for instructors to have a general understanding

> ### Did you know?
> Many Japanese desk workers stand up every hour to stretch. This can stretch the hip flexor muscles, which if left in a shortened seated position all day can contribute to back pain.

of this area therefore a simple description of the types of stretches listed earlier follows below.

Static

This is when a stretch is performed and held for a period of time at a point of mild tension (not pain). The point of tension is a subjective perception (what the person feels) and is thought to reduce as the person gets used to stretching. If a static stretch is held for long enough, this tension usually subsides and the stretch can be taken further if required. If a partner or another group of muscles assists in the stretching process it is called an active stretch. If there is no assistance in the stretch it is called a passive stretch.

Dynamic

This relates to stretching in motion where an agonist muscle is contracted to stretch an antagonist muscle (the muscle doing the work contracts to stretch the opposite muscle). This type of stretching is usually carried out in a slow and controlled manner in order to minimise the risk of injury caused by uncontrolled or rapid movements and to mimic the types of movement that may be used in the exercises used in the same session.

Ballistic

This is where bouncing movements are caused by momentum or gravity. This type of stretching is usually carried out by athletes who are familiar with this type of stretching. As there is little control of the movement through muscular contraction there is a greater potential for risk of injury.

PNF

The term PNF is otherwise known as 'proprioceptive neuromuscular facilitation' (you can see why it is shortened to PNF!). This is a type of partner assisted stretching, usually carried out on tight or injured muscles. There is usually a degree of training associated with this type of stretching and as such it should only be performed by those who are qualified to do so. Contract-relax-antagonist-contract (CRAC) is another form of this type of stretching.

It is impossible for any individual to have what can be considered as optimum flexibility in all joints as the demands of people's everyday lives are so different. It is important, therefore, to identify why particular flexibility is needed due to the effects of the hormone relaxin increasing flexibility anyway. Leading up to pregnancy it might be useful to think of an individual's needs in terms of flexibility especially if they take part in any particular sports or activities. The exercise in the 'Try this!' box will help you think about flexibility needs.

Stability

Because of the hormonal effects on flexibility during pregnancy it is essential for instructors to have some understanding of the term 'stability'. Stability is in effect the opposite of flexibility as it refers to how joints can be kept in a stable position to do the job for which they were designed. For instance, the shoulder joint is much more flex-

Try this!

Place a tick in the box that is relevant to each sport in terms of importance of flexibility.

	Low	Medium	High
Aerobics		✔	
Dancing			
Netball			
Running/jogging			
Darts			
Snooker			
Cycling			
Badminton			
Tennis			
Archery	✔		
Gymnastics			✔
Martial arts			

ible than the hip joint because, although they are both classed as synovial ball and socket joints, the hip joint is a much deeper joint than the shoulder joint. It has evolved this way because the hip joint requires a great deal more stability than the shoulder joint for everyday use and the shoulder joint requires a greater range of motion and flexibility to move than the hip joint.

Flexibility beyond a 'normal' range of motion may be useful or necessary in certain circumstances such as childbirth, but it should be remembered that the muscular system is one of three main systems that contribute to joint stability as shown in figure 12.8. It is generally agreed that all three systems play an important role in the prevention

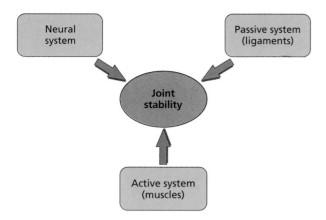

Figure 12.8 Systems contributing to overall joint stability

- Static balance: This simply means to maintain equilibrium (balance) in a stationary position.
- Dynamic balance: This means to maintain equilibrium (balance) while in motion.

The ability of an individual to be able to balance is absolutely fundamental to any effective movement, not just in a sporting context but in everyday life and in particular for women who are pregnant. For example, when walking, jogging or running in a straight line, balance is absolutely crucial for effective foot placement, body control and reduction of 'core' movement. For this reason, balance is also often described as 'control of the centre of mass' because if we are in control of our centre of mass then we are in a balanced and stable position.

Due to the postural changes associated with pregnancy, balance becomes an even more crucial component of fitness as the passive system (ligaments) becomes less able to contribute to joint stability. Although a complex area, there are systems in the body that contribute to balance such as proprioception, visual and vestibular systems which are considered to be the main systems.

Proprioception system

Located in all of the joints around the body are tiny sensors known as 'proprioceptors'. These sensors are able to detect joint position then relay

of joint injury as a result of instability, however, as ligament tissue is prone to tearing (see page 29), the muscular system is often required to provide an additional or greater amount of stability for joints, especially during dynamic movements. If an individual's flexibility is considered to be greater than the normal range-of-motion (hyper flexibility), joint stability may be found to be lacking or reduced, resulting in a variety of conditions or joint injury. Conversely, where the flexibility of an individual is considered to be less than the normal range (hypo-flexibility), injury such as muscle strain can occur.

BALANCE

Generally speaking there are two types or categories of balance; 'static balance' and 'dynamic balance'. It has been shown that both of these types of balance can be developed with the correct type of training, especially in young children. Even though there are many definitions, the following can be used for the purpose of simplicity:

What does this term mean?

Proprioceptors are tiny sensors in the body that detect tension in tendons. This information can then be used to work out the position of joints, which is then relayed to the brain.

this information to the brain on a constant basis so that the position of the limbs etc. is regularly updated for balance purposes. For instance, if you go over on your ankle, the proprioceptors around the joint would send information to the brain to say that the ankle joint was in a potentially dangerous position. In response to this information the brain would stimulate the necessary leg muscles to try and regain balance before the injury occurred.

During pregnancy and for a period of time afterwards, this system is less effective due to the effects of the hormone relaxin on the ligaments.

Visual system

Most of our balance information comes from what we see. In other words, this is our visual referencing system. Our eyes continually use the objects around us to determine our balance and the following example can illustrate how much we rely on this.

> Have you ever been running on a treadmill then when it stops, you feel like you are still moving or you feel off balance?
>
> This is because when you walk or run, the image on the retina from objects around you changes size as you get nearer or further away and over the years your brain learns to expect this. Running on a treadmill causes confusion for the brain because the objects around you don't change size!

Vestibular system

Within the inner ear there are a series of canals filled with fluid. The canals are lined with tiny hairs and if we move in any direction the fluid flows over the tiny hairs, which provides information to the brain that we are moving (in a particular direction). This is why if you ever get an ear infection or a condition such as vertigo or vestibular neuritis, your balance can be affected. An instructor should pay particular attention to a client who has an inner ear infection as both their proprioception and vestibular systems will be compromised and as pregnancy also affects balance, there may be additional issues.

As can be seen, the brain relies upon sources of information from the eyes, the ears and proprioceptors for balance purposes. Through regular training of these systems, the ability to perform balance skills usually becomes more effective. In addition, it is thought that the brain becomes better able to interpret the balance information from the various systems so that it can make the appropriate movement response. The communication system within the body (made up of nerves) is developed during movement skills training. The 'neural networks' within the brain and nervous system become more extensive as more and more neural links are created through repetition of movement skills. Introducing complex movements increases balance requirements. The ability to land, accelerate, change direction and decelerate, requires advanced balance skills. A training programme, therefore, should follow a logical progression in relation to the complexity of skills to be performed that will allow the development of balance skills. It is also advised that balance skills be introduced as far in advance of conception as possible in order to minimise the reduced effect of the proprioceptive system during pregnancy.

EXERCISE SELECTION

KEY POINTS

- There are many cardiovascular machines that are suitable in different ways, therefore instructors are advised to familiarise themselves with all machines prior to selection and client induction.
- The cycle, the stepper and rowing machines are considered to be non-impact machines that can be used for those individuals wishing to avoid any impact on the joints.
- Resistance exercises can be broadly categorised into two subclassifications or groups. These groups are known as 'stabilisation' and 'mobilisation' exercises for which there are specific muscle groups related to each.
- Resistance machines are not the most functional way to train for strength or endurance, however they do minimise the risk of incorrect technique and provide support for the back.
- Free weights do require correct posture and good core stability to be maintained, which may be difficult in later stages of pregnancy.
- There is a wide range of possible group exercise classes that the pregnant woman may choose to attend but instructors must consider the suitability of each specific to their client.
- If an individual does have a pre-existing or pregnancy-induced medical condition then it is important for the instructor to work closely with the primary antenatal care provider to ensure that any activity is safe for the mother-to-be and the foetus.
- It is not considered to be appropriate to progress exercise during pregnancy. In most cases there will be some regression (in terms of the volume and intensity of the exercise) as the pregnancy progresses.

SELECTION OF EXERCISES DURING PREGNANCY

It is often difficult when selecting the types of exercise activities that are suitable during the pregnancy period. Although no definitive list exists, table 13.1 gives a suggestion of those activities that are thought to be suitable, those that are not suitable and those to which caution should be applied.

When deciding which gym-based exercises are appropriate for clients, it should help the instructor to address the areas related to the components of fitness, such as cardiovascular,

Table 13.1	Exercise activity suitability during pregnancy			
Type	**Yes**	**No**	**Caution**	**Comments**
Aerobics			✓	Low impact, low intensity only
Gym – CV	✓			Reduce intensity as pregnancy progresses
Gym – MSE	✓			Reduce resistance as pregnancy progresses
Aqua	✓			Ante natal specific recommended
Yoga or Pilates			✓	Reduce range/intensity, no supine work after 20 weeks, ante natal specific recommended
Running			✓	Reduce distance/speed as pregnancy progresses, jogging/walking as alternatives

muscular strength and endurance, flexibility and balance. The instructor should also be aware that exercise guidelines in relation to frequency, intensity, timing and type should be followed.

CARDIOVASCULAR

Today there are many cardiovascular machines that are available for selection, therefore instructors are advised to familiarise themselves with all

Table 13.2	Treadmill
Suitability	The treadmill can be used for both walking and running but is associated with greater impact on the joints than other cardiovascular machines. It is suitable throughout pregnancy for most healthy clients.
Intensity	Beginners should stick to walking through all three trimesters. Experienced runners may wish to continue to run in trimester one and it is recommended that they slow intensity to a light jog in trimester two and to a brisk walk in trimester three.
Foot action	A heel-toe action should be encouraged at walking and jogging pace as this will help to absorb the shock of impact. At speeds around 8mph, the client should be encouraged to use a mid foot strike as this will help to eliminate the braking effect.
Arm action	The most efficient way to swing the arms is with a 90-degree angle at the elbows and the arms swinging close to the side of the body. Try to keep the shoulders relaxed and down at all times. Be aware that moderate to vigorous arm action may be uncomfortable for the breasts, particularly throughout trimesters two and three.
Posture	Encourage the client to maintain a neutral spine with only a slight lean forward, which will increase slightly as the treadmill is inclined.
Considerations	Beginners may feel unstable when a treadmill comes to a stop and this can cause unsteadiness for a short period (see information on balance, page 103).

machines prior to selection and client induction. For example, before a client begins a programme of exercise, it is necessary that they are familiar with the equipment they are going to use. Some of the most common cardiovascular machines are the treadmill, cycle, stepper/cross trainer and rower. An explanation of each is given in tables 13.2 to 13.10.

Table 13.3	Upright cycle
Suitability	There is no impact associated with using the cycle so it is recommended throughout pregnancy. It is also ideal as an exercise modality for obese or arthritic clients who need to reduce the amount of impact to the joints. If the client experiences discomfort in the genital area the seat may be uncomfortable.
Intensity pedal speed (cadence/rpm)	Actual pedal speed depends on the preference of the client. Most people prefer to pedal between 50 and 80rpm (revs/minute) although speeds should be reduced in the second and third trimesters of pregnancy.
Seat height	Seat height can affect the range of motion and speed of the legs so it is important to make sure that the seat is level with the hip joint of the client when standing next to the cycle. With the client on the cycle and the feet flat in the pedals, the knee should have a slight bend at the furthest point of the rotation. However, during pregnancy the seat may need to be lower to minimise rocking of the pelvis and extension at the knee joint.
Posture	Encourage an upright posture with neutral spine at all times.

Table 13.4	Recumbent cycle
Suitability	There is no impact associated with using the recumbent cycle so it is suitable throughout pregnancy. However, as the uterus enlarges it may not be possible for the mother-to-be to cycle with the knees in alignment, which may lead to hip abduction and therefore be uncomfortable in the later parts of trimesters two and three.
Intensity pedal speed (cadence/rpm)	Actual pedal speed depends on the preference of the client. Most people prefer to pedal between 50 and 80rpm although speeds and levels should be reduced in the second and third trimesters of pregnancy.
Seat position	As the seat position can affect the range of motion and speed of the legs, it is important to make sure that the seat is positioned so that the knee has a slight bend at the furthest point of the rotation when the client is on the cycle with the feet flat in the pedals.
Posture	Encourage clients not to press the back flat into the seat and to try and maintain a neutral spine. The use of a rolled towel should help this.

Table 13.5	Stepper
Suitability	The stepper is suitable for the first and early second trimesters and can be used later in pregnancy if pelvic alignment is maintained. If any pelvic pain is experienced this machine should not be used.
Intensity	Intensity levels should be gradually reduced through the pregnancy and by trimester three a maximum of 10-minute periods is advised.
Action	Maintain a position with the shoulder, hip and heel in line (when viewed from the side) and keep the pelvis in alignment. Make sure the full range of movement is used (usually at least 6–8in).
Posture	Maintain an upright posture with a neutral spine at all times.

Table 13.6	Cross trainer/elliptical trainer
Suitability	The cross trainer is low impact so suitable through pregnancy, particularly for those who are already experienced in its use, and provided pelvic alignment can be maintained.
Intensity	Select a speed that is comfortable for the client. As the level on the step machine is increased, the resistance of the pedals will decrease which means that the client will need to increase the speed. Use the leg action only for warming up or cooling down and for a workout in trimester three.
Range of motion	With the whole of the foot placed on the step, encourage a full range of motion that is just before the end range of the machine. Reduce stride length if necessary for pelvic comfort in mid to late pregnancy.
Action	As the leg rises during the stepping action, the heel of the same leg should rise slightly off the pedal and return to the pedal as the leg goes down to mimic actual stepping motion. This helps to promote blood flow round the body as a result of the calf muscle squeezing (venous return).
Posture	Encourage the client to hold the handles to the side of the body and not out in front. This will enable the client to maintain an upright posture with neutral spine.

Table 13.7	Arc trainer/walker/glider
Suitability	This type of machine is suitable during the first trimester and early second trimester. As knees remain straight throughout the full range of movement it is likely to cause the pelvis to rock, which makes it difficult to keep pelvic alignment. Therefore this machine is not suitable after about 18–20 weeks.
Intensity	This can be a moderate to vigorous intensity machine due to arm and leg action so intensity should be kept low while it is being used.
Posture	Maintain an upright posture with a neutral spine and a slight bend in the knee.

Table 13.8	Rower
Suitability	As a low Impact machine, the rower is suitable through pregnancy. However, it may be difficult to get on and off the lower versions in later pregnancy and the growing abdominal bulk may also prevent correct technique or place stress on the lower back. As soon as the thighs start to touch the abdomen or the hips abduct it is time to stop!
Intensity	Intensity levels will need to decrease gradually during pregnancy.
Action	**Start position (catch):** With the feet secured in the straps and the knees bent, hold the handle with a pronated grip (overhand) with the arms out straight and a slight bend at the elbows. Keep the wrists straight. The back should be in an upright neutral position. **Drive:** Initiate the drive phase with legs pushing out. As the legs are almost at full stretch, pull the handle into the abdomen area. **Recovery:** The arms must extend fully before the legs bend to allow the body to come back to the start position. The recovery phase should be twice as long as the drive phase.
Posture	Maintain an upright posture with a neutral spine and avoid leaning too far back during the drive.

Table 13.9	Upper body ergometer/arm bike
Suitability	This type of machine utilises only the upper body and there is a risk that heart rate and blood pressure levels may be increased beyond those recommended by the Royal College of Obstetricians and Gynaecologists. However it may be the only option for a client who has limited or no lower body mobility or function and in such cases expert advice should be sought.

Table 13.10	Other CV machines (e.g. Wave, VersaClimber, ski track, etc.)
Suitability	These machines are only suitable for those who are experienced in their use and only during the first trimester and early part of the second trimester. If they are used as part of a sport conditioning/maintenance programme, expert advice should be sought.

Summary for cardiovascular machine training

As there is no impact associated with any exercise related to the use of either type of cycle, they can be used as an exercise modality for those individuals who need to reduce the amount of impact to the joints. This could be in cases such as obese or arthritic individuals. As with the treadmill, cycles can be used for either aerobic or anaerobic conditioning depending on the intensity that the exercise is performed at. As for the treadmill, it can be used for both walking and running but instructors should note that it is also associated with greater impact on the joints than any other of the cardiovascular machines. Like the cycle, the stepper and rowing machines are also considered

Table 13.11	Overview of cardiovascular machine appropriateness		
Machine	**Trimester one**	**Trimester two**	**Trimester three**
Treadmill	Yes – walking, jogging and running as appropriate	Yes – walking and light jogging only	Yes – walking recommended
Upright bike	Yes	Yes	Yes
Recumbent bike	Yes	Yes – caution due to the size of the abdomen and need to avoid hip abduction	
Cross/elliptical trainer	Yes	Possible if pelvic alignment is good, but reduce intensity	Possible with legs only and only if pelvic alignment is good
Stepper	Yes	Caution: Technique needs to be excellent and intensity should be low	
Arc trainer/glider	Yes	Not recommended due to pelvic action	
Rower	Yes	Caution: Due to the size of the abdomen and need to avoid hip abduction; should be low intensity only	
Arm bike	Only for those with low body mobility issues and no hypertension		

to be non-impact machines that can be used for those individuals wishing to avoid any impact on the joints, however, it is important to remember that it has often been demonstrated that rowing can place a greater amount of stress on the lower back muscles than any other method of cardiovascular exercise.

Finally, as each trimester can be associated with a variety of different potential problems in relation to pregnancy, table 13.11 gives an overview of the guidelines for appropriateness as recommended by the authors.

In terms of showing the client how to use the cardiovascular machines correctly, the IDEA method is one of the most common approaches used in the health and fitness industry (please refer to chapter 9, page 78, for a full explanation of this particular method of instruction).

MUSCULAR STRENGTH AND ENDURANCE

In order to prepare the body for the demands of pregnancy and the postnatal period to follow, there is a vast number of resistance-type exercises that the instructor can choose from (depending on the goals of the client), as it has been shown that low-to-moderate intensity strength training programmes during pregnancy can be safe and efficacious for pregnant women (O'Connor et al 1990).

In terms of muscular strength and endurance (see page 96 for definitions of these terms), exercises can be broadly categorised into two subclassifications or groups. These groups are known as 'stabilisation' and 'mobilisation' exercises. They are categorised in this way due to the particular daily demands (referred to as 'activities of daily living') of the muscle groups and what function they were specifically designed to carry out. Table

Table 13.12	Typical muscle groups associated with stabilisation and mobilisation
Stabilisation muscles	**Mobilisation muscles**
Spinal stabilisation:	Spinal mobilisation:
• Transversus abdominis (TA)	• Rectus abdominis (RA)
• Multifidis	• Erector spinae
• Internal obliques	• External obliques
• Quadratus lumborum	
• Diaphragm	
• Pelvic floor	
Shoulder/scapula stabilisation:	Shoulder mobilisation:
• Teres major	• Anterior deltoid
• Teres minor	• Posterior deltoid
• Infraspinatus	• Pectoralis major
• Supraspinatus	• Latissimus dorsi
• Serratus anterior	• Trapezius
• Rhomboids	• Triceps brachii
	• Biceps brachii
Hip stabilisation:	Hip mobilisation:
• Piriformis	• Gluteus maximus
• Gluteus medius	• Hamstrings
• Gluteus minimis	• Quadriceps
• Adductor longus	
• Adductor brevis	
• Adductor magnus	
• Pectinius	
• Gracilis	
• Deep hip rotators	

13.12 shows the muscle groups that generally fit into the two categories (even though this is not an exclusive list) and covers the shoulder, spine and hip areas as these are the joints in the body that require the greatest amount of stabilisation. For example, the hip and shoulder joints are classed as freely moveable joints (synovial joints) and the spine is a series of slightly moveable interlocking joints that often has to withstand large amounts of force.

Stabilisation and mobilisation

In simple terms, stabilisation relates to maintaining the stability of all joints in the body and in particular the spine, shoulder and hip joints. In order to do so, the muscles that are responsible for this role must function correctly so that other muscles that are responsible for movement (mobilisation) are able to perform their function correctly. Unfortunately, it is quite common that as a result of joint stabilising muscles becoming weaker, and in some cases not activating correctly, other muscles that are usually associated with movement tasks have to take on the role of stabilisation. This often leads to weakness and can eventually cause muscle, tendon or ligament injury, especially in cases where the speed of a movement is increased. This will in turn increase the possibility of injury due to the greater demand for stabilisation.

Because stabilisation is associated with endurance-type activity, muscles that stabilise (stabilisers) are often found to have a high percentage of Type 1 slow-twitch fibres. These muscles are sometimes referred to as 'tonic' muscles. If stabilisers are working correctly, muscles known as 'mobilisers' are able to carry out their role of providing movement. These muscles are usually required to provide a short-term role (phasic) and are often found to have more fast-twitch fibres and be more superficial (closer to the surface) than the deep stabiliser muscles. One of the reasons why it is important to distinguish between stabilising and mobilising exercises is that they are often trained to perform the opposite role that they were designed for. For example, the rectus abdominis is predominantly a fast-twitch muscle close to the surface of the body and is normally active in strength or explosive tasks (phasic role) such as running and jumping where the legs come towards the torso (spinal flexion). However, the rectus abdominis is often trained using sit-up-type exercises that are performed repetitively as in an endurance-type capacity (tonic). This type of regular exercise often has the effect of weakening the spinal stabiliser muscles as they are no longer used for the task of stabilisation as the rectus abdominis has taken on this role. This 'reversal' of roles is commonplace in exercise programmes not just for the rectus abdominis but for many different muscles within the body. It should be noted however, that during pregnancy the role of the rectus abdominis as a fast-twitch mobiliser is diminished greatly, as the movements explained previously are not necessarily required and the strength of the muscle can reduce quite significantly. For this reason it is important that the stabiliser muscles are as strong as they can be to support the postural changes that will occur.

Equipment for muscular strength and endurance training

Resistance machines are not the most functional way to train for strength or endurance, however they do minimise the risk of incorrect tech-

Table 13.13	Overview of resistance guidelines	
Trimester one	**Trimester two**	**Trimester three**
Continue as normal provided the client is comfortable to do so. Avoid Valsalva manoeuvre (forced exhalation with nose and mouth are closed).	Reduce resistance levels by 5% or more of pre-pregnancy levels in the first half of this trimester, and by a further 5–10% or more during the second trimester.	Reduce resistance by a further 5–10% or more of pre-pregnancy levels. Levels should be approximately 70% of pre-pregnancy levels by the end of this trimester.

Adapted from Baker (2006)

Table 13.14	Recommended muscular strength and endurance exercises through pregnancy	
Exercise	**Function/purpose**	**Alternative/comments**
Squats Lunges	To build strength/endurance in the leg muscles and help with lifting techniques	Leg press: May be uncomfortable after the first trimester
Calf raises	Maintain venous return; help with balance	Seated calf raises
Lat pulldown Seated row	Help maintain posture; build strength in the upper back to help with lifting	Cable machines
Bent over row		Single arm row
Chest press	Maintain strength in the chest	Resistance band press
Shoulder press/ lateral raise	Maintain strength/endurance in the shoulder muscles. Caution: Shoulder press not suitable after the first trimester due to overhead movement	Lateral/front raises more appropriate in trimesters two and three
Triceps extension/ pushdown	Maintain strength in the triceps	Resistance band press
Biceps curl	Maintain strength in the biceps	Dumbbell curls
Internal/external shoulder rotations	Maintain posture and avoid kyphosis	Dumb waiter with resistance band

nique and provide support for the back. In later stages of pregnancy there may be issues with abdomen and breast size and/or tenderness. Although a more effective way to train muscles, free weights do require correct posture and good core stability to be maintained, which may be difficult in later stages of pregnancy. Resistance bands are very suitable throughout pregnancy and can be used easily and effectively in group sessions or one to one. They are also useful for chair based sessions.

Exercise selection

In terms of the selection of exercises for muscular strength and endurance, chapter 14 provides a range that deal with the muscles that stabilise the hip, shoulder and spine joints. The muscles that are responsible for the stabilisation of each joint can be seen in table 13.12. Some of the spinal stabilisation exercises require the use of a stability

ball and it is recommended that instructors are experienced in this area prior to delivering these exercises. If using a stability ball, consideration must be given to the balance and proprioceptive ability of the client.

Other exercises that are recommended for pregnant women focus on posture, functional ability and preparation for the activities associated with having babies and children. Key exercises are included in table 13.14 and the focus should be on a whole-body approach.

An experienced instructor will be able to adapt other exercises for a pregnant client and must be aware of functional and pregnancy-related limitations and ensure safe and effective performance at all times.

GROUP EXERCISE CLASSES

There are now many types of group exercise sessions available and it is likely that a pregnant

Try this!

Identify the suitability of the following types of session during pregnancy.

Type	Yes	No	Cautions	Alternative
Exercise to music				
Gym				
Aqua				
Yoga				
Pilates				
Outdoor				
Combat classes				
Group indoor cycling				

client will wish to continue in her regular class for as long as possible. It is not unheard of for a woman to continue with her aerobics right up to birth, but it does require considerable knowledge on the part of the instructor to ensure it is safe for her to do so. It is recommended that all instructors hold a specific Ante- and Postnatal qualification if working with pregnant women on a regular basis.

As there is a wide range of possible group exercise classes that the pregnant woman may choose to attend, table 13.15 considers the suitability and intensity levels, and comments on a range of group exercise modalities.

Table 13.15	Group exercise classes and their suitability
Aerobics	
Suitability	Low-impact and low-intensity classes are suitable in the first trimester, however after 16 weeks supine lying is to be avoided and intensity will need to be reduced, so a dedicated antenatal class is a preferred option after this time.
Intensity	• During pregnancy the resting heart rate may be 10–15bpm above non-pregnant states so the intensity of the session, including warm-up and cool down, will need to be lowered. • Core temperature is higher during pregnancy so all elements of the session must progress or reduce in intensity gradually. The warm-up should be shorter but still progress gradually.
Comments	Balance may be affected so quick changes of direction, cueing or impact need to be adapted.
Step	
Suitability	Not recommended for newcomers to exercise. Regular step participants may be able to continue provided the instructor is qualified to work in this area, class intensity is reduced and the height of the step is lowered.
Intensity	• Can be intense so a beginner class may be more suitable during pregnancy. • Participants should reduce the height of the step, so that by the end it should be no more than the step box alone.
Comments	• Complex choreography may be harder for pregnant women to follow and there is a risk of tripping with moves over or around the step. • Correct technique is important to avoid joint impact. • Pelvic alignment is important so if it is compromised, recommend a different class.

Body conditioning/Legs, Bums, Tums

Suitability	Standing or seated sessions only after 16th week of pregnancy.
Intensity	Resistance must be gradually reduced (see gym section above) throughout pregnancy and movements must be controlled.
Comments	Provided supine or prone lying is avoided and resistance and intensity are reduced gradually this type of session may be continued.

Circuits

Suitability	Not recommended for newcomers to exercise. Regular circuit-goers can continue as long as they reduce intensity at cardiovascular stations and weight at muscular strength/endurance stations. Pelvic alignment should be maintained.
Intensity	• Ensure a lower intensity to avoid overheating and a reduced range of movement to protect joints. • Avoid any prone or supine stations after the 16th week of pregnancy.
Comments	• Quick changes may affect balance. • Recommend a dedicated antenatal circuit.

Studio resistance

Suitability	• A low-impact session so may be suitable throughout pregnancy if well adapted and if the woman is already an experienced participant in this type of class. • No supine work after 16 weeks and intensity should be reduced as pregnancy progresses.
Intensity	• Resistance, repetitions and rate all need to be reduced during pregnancy. Towards the end of trimester three these should be at approximately 70% of pre-pregnancy levels. • Rest must be increased as pregnancy progresses.
Comments	Consider a specific antenatal 'toning' session instead.

Combat

Suitability	• Combat or martial arts-style sessions are generally high intensity and high impact so are not suitable during pregnancy. • Additionally, the joints may work through a larger range, or be affected by momentum and impact, none of which are suitable during pregnancy. • A further consideration is that it is hard to maintain good pelvic alignment for some of the moves.

Latin (including Zumba™)

Suitability	• The high intensity, fast pace and excessive torso and pelvic movements which are a feature of this type of session are not recommended during pregnancy, particularly for beginners. • If a client is keen to continue in these classes they must be led by an instructor who holds a full Level 3 Ante- and Postnatal qualification and who has undergone specific training in adapting this type of session for pregnant women.

Group indoor cycling

Suitability	• Only suitable for those experienced in this type of class and with a low risk pregnancy due to the intensity of the session. • Specific antenatal indoor cycling classes are available and these would be more appropriate than mainstream classes.
Intensity	Intensity in group indoor cycling sessions is usually much too high for a pregnant woman so either use minimal resistance or reduce speed.
Comments	• Posture should be correct at all times, avoiding a forward lean or curved spine. • Pelvic alignment is important as excessive rocking may lead to pain in the pelvic area.

Yoga

Suitability	• Specific antenatal yoga sessions with an appropriately trained instructor are suitable during pregnancy. • Due to the effects of relaxin on the joints other types of yoga cannot be recommended, so-called 'hot' yoga and dynamic yoga are **not** suitable at any stage of pregnancy due to overheating and rapid changes of position.
Intensity	• Movements may need to be slower and range of movement decreased to avoid joint issues. • Avoid developmental stretching and limit stretches to under 30 seconds. • Avoid wide leg postures and holding postures that stress the pelvis for longer than 30 seconds. • Inversions are not appropriate during pregnancy.
Comments	Instructors should undergo specific training in yoga for pregnancy.

Pilates

Suitability	• Pilates is considered to be safe during trimester one. After the 16th week of pregnancy any exercise that places stress on the rectus abdominis or oblique muscles should be discontinued to minimise the risk of diastasis recti.
	• Supine and prone work should also be avoided after this time to avoid supine hypotension and minimise discomfort.
	• All fours and side-lying positions are appropriate; however cushions may be needed under the knees and bump!
	• Sit back up after each set of exercises performed on all fours and encourage wrist mobility to avoid problems with carpal tunnel syndrome.
	• Avoid wide leg positions after the first trimester to minimise pelvic discomfort.
Intensity	Pilates is a low-intensity activity so no modifications are necessary other than those mentioned above and the following considerations:
	• Reduce the number of reps as pregnancy progresses.
	• Reduce range of movement and length of levers.
	• Omit lumbar extensor concentric work to avoid increasing lumbar lordosis.
Comments	Instructors should undergo specific training in Pilates for pregnancy to ensure safe and effective sessions.

Aqua

Suitability	Suitable throughout pregnancy.
Intensity	Intensity is usually appropriate, however pool temperature may need to be adjusted to avoid cooling down or overheating.
Comments	• Instructors should undergo specific aqua natal training.
	• Many classes are led by a qualified instructor in conjunction with a practising midwife and these are recommended, particularly for women during their first pregnancy who may not know how their body will respond to exercise, or who are nervous about activity.

Table 13.16 provides a summary of the authors' recommendations in relation to the suitability of each modality broken down into each particular trimester.

The recommendations in relation to exercises discussed in this chapter are specific to those pregnant women who have no pre-existing or pregnancy-induced medical conditions (see chapter 4 for more information). If an individual does, however, have any of the conditions, then it is important for the instructor to work closely with the primary antenatal care provider to ensure that any activity is safe for the mother-to-be and the foetus.

In terms of the progression of any of the exercises within the group environment, this is not considered to be appropriate during pregnancy. In most cases there will be some regression (in terms of the volume and intensity of the exercise) as the pregnancy progresses.

Table 13.16	Overview of group exercise classes		
Type	**Trimester one**	**Trimester two**	**Trimester three**
Aerobics	Yes	Caution: Low impact only, reduce intensity	
Step	Caution: Lower height of step and intensity, maintain pelvic alignment		Not recommended
Legs, Bums, Tums	Yes	Caution: Reduce intensity, no supine work	
Circuits	Yes – reduce intensity		Caution
Studio resistance/ body pump	Caution	Caution: No supine work and reduce resistance used to approx. 70% of pre-pregnancy loads	
Combat	Not recommended	Not recommended	Not recommended
Latin (Zumba™)	Caution – reduce intensity and pelvic movements	Not recommended	Not recommended
Group cycling	Caution – reduce resistance and intensity	Not recommended – no resistance and very low intensity only; incorporate rest breaks	
Yoga	Caution	Antenatal specific – **no hot yoga**	
Pilates	Yes	Antenatal specific – **avoid supine work**	
Aqua	Yes	Yes, ideally antenatal specific	

As the range of activities that a pregnant woman can participate in is vast, it is impossible to give guidelines relating to them all. It is, however, worth summarising brief guidelines related to some of the more common possibilities such as those in table 13.17.

Type	Trimester one	Trimester two	Trimester three
Table 13.17	**Guidelines related to other activities and sports**		
Walking	Yes	Yes	Yes
Running or jogging	Yes, if experienced	Yes, if experienced, although reduce distance and intensity	Yes, but reduce distance to 2 miles a day and reduce pace
Cycling	Yes	• Balance, coordination issues may result in falls • Intensity needs to be reduced	
Swimming	Yes	Yes, however breaststroke may cause discomfort on pubic symphysis and lumbar spine	
Diving	• Risk of physical trauma from high diving • Scuba diving not recommended		
Climbing	• Not recommended due to risk of falling • Grip may be compromised by carpal tunnel syndrome		
Horse riding	Not recommended due to risk of falling		
Skiing	Experienced skiers may continue, however balance and coordination issues may increase the risk of falling		
Contact sports	Not recommended due to risk of direct impact (person, equipment) and risk of falling		
Water sports	Not recommended due to risk of falling, impact with water or possibility of air embolism		
Gymnastics	Not recommended due to effects of relaxin on connective tissue and risk of falling		

INSTRUCTING EXERCISE DURING PREGNANCY

Fitness instructors who continue to teach classes while pregnant themselves should also follow the recommendations above and protect their own health.

- Demonstrations need to be impact free and range should be reduced.
- Intensity should be kept low to avoid over-heating or joint issues.
- Focus more on observation and correction of participants than on your own performance and always keep within a comfortable intensity.

- The number of classes taught may need to be reduced if fatigue is increased.

For most instructors the growing abdomen and their own health will naturally slow them down, and provided they apply the above guidelines to themselves as well as to clients, there is no reason why they should not continue to teach through their pregnancy. However, it is important to keep the relevant health care providers aware of the number and type of classes involved, and if they advise reducing or stopping the number of classes, this should be heeded.

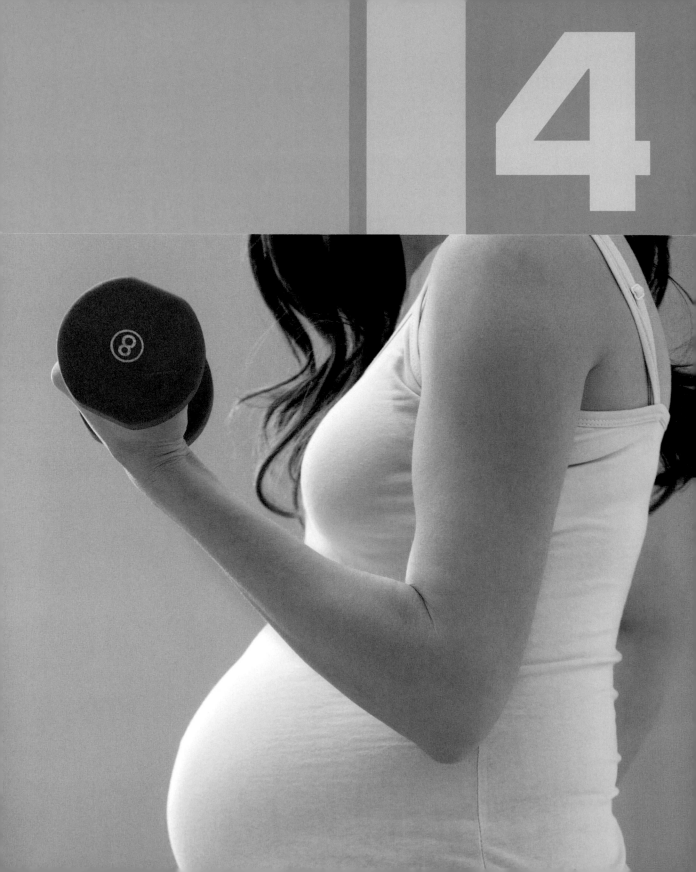

PART **FOUR**

THE EXERCISES

EXERCISING DURING PREGNANCY

14

INTRODUCTION

The main aim of activity during pregnancy is to maintain a reasonable level of fitness and to promote good posture, in particular helping to avoid development or worsening of the typical kyphotic and lordotic postures that are associated with pregnancy. The exercises that are described in this chapter were chosen as they have proved to be beneficial during pregnancy, however there are cautions given where an exercise may be unsuitable in the second or third trimesters and these should be adhered to. At all times the comfort and confidence of the mother-to-be must be considered, so if she feels uncomfortable with any particular exercise or position, adaptations should be made.

The length and intensity of the session needs to be planned with the client in mind. Beginners to activity will need to start at a low intensity, which will remain at a relatively low level throughout the pregnancy. Warm-ups should progress gradually to an RPE of 2–3 on the modified scale while intensity in the main activity should not exceed 5 or 6. Cool-downs are intended to return the body to a pre-exercise state so will gradually lower in intensity until the client is feeling 'normal'. The length of the session should be shorter to accom-

modate lower fitness and skill levels – anywhere from 30–45 minutes would be appropriate. More experienced exercisers can work to a higher level, tapering the intensity down as the pregnancy progresses. The length of the session may be up to 60 minutes, however it is recommended that this reduces as the pregnancy progresses.

Antenatal group exercise sessions normally have participants with a mix of fitness levels and pregnancy duration which will need to be taken into consideration when planning and this is not easy. A low intensity, simpler and shorter session may be frustrating for those who are regular class participants, while a moderate intensity session with more complex choreography will be off-putting for the less experienced or new exercisers. It is therefore important to have a range of alternatives planned for the session and as the regulars are likely to be able to follow the choreography and monitor their own intensity the instructor should always stay with the less fit or experienced exercisers to make sure they are comfortable – while keeping an eye on the regulars to make sure they are not overdoing it! An alternative may be to offer different classes for beginners or regulars to provide the most appropriate environment for all.

Circuit approaches work well as stations can be adapted for all levels and durations of pregnancy and the instructor can observe and monitor easily. If an instructor does not hold a specific circuit qualification there are general and pregnancy-specific modules and workshops available which improve knowledge and skills to help with this type of session. One-to-one sessions, whether gym based or personal training sessions, are easier to plan as the fitness and skill levels of the client will be known and can be adapted as necessary.

STRETCHING EXERCISES

Exercise 14.1 Seated hamstring stretch

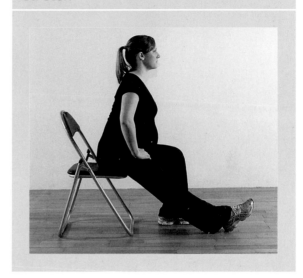

Major muscles used
Hamstrings

Action
- Sit on a stable chair with the bottom towards the front of the chair. Keep the spine in a neutral position.
- Take one leg out in front with the knee straight but not forced, and relax the foot.
- Lean forward making sure to pivot from the hip and keep the spine in a neutral position.
- Take the stretch only as far as is comfortable.

Awareness points
Maintain a normal lumbar curve at all times.

Alternatives
Standing hamstring stretch

Exercise 14.2 Seated chest stretch

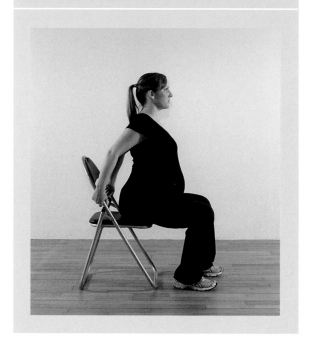

Exercise 14.3 Seated lat stretch

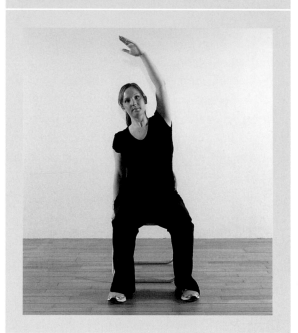

Major muscles used

Pectoralis major

Action

- Sit on a stable chair with the bottom towards the front of the chair. Keep the spine in a neutral position.
- Outwardly rotate the arms and take the hands behind and place on the lower back or on the chair back.
- Sit tall and lean slightly forward until a comfortable stretch is felt across the chest.

Awareness points

Maintain a normal lumbar curve at all times.

Alternatives

Standing chest press, one arm chest press

Major muscles used

Latissimus Dorsi

Action

- Sit on a stable chair with the bottom towards the front of the chair. Keep the spine in a neutral position.
- Place one hand on the chair seat and raise the other hand overhead.
- Lengthen the arm up towards the ceiling and lean slightly over until a comfortable stretch is felt.

Awareness points

Maintain a normal lumbar curve at all times.

Alternatives

Standing lat stretch

Exercise 14.4 Seated adductor stretch

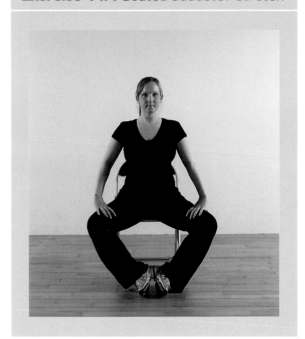

Major muscles used
Adductors

Action
- Sit on a stable chair with the bottom towards the front of the chair. Keep the spine in a neutral position.
- Place the feet together and on their sides.
- Take the knees out and press gently until a comfortable stretch is felt.

Awareness points
Maintain a normal lumbar curve at all times.

Alternatives
Standing adductor stretch

Exercise 14.5 Standing quad stretch

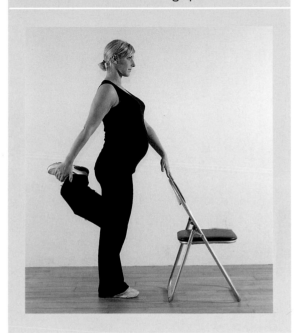

Major muscles used
Quadriceps, hip flexors

Action
- Stand next to a stable support. Keep the spine in a neutral position.
- Shift the weight onto one leg and lift the other foot up behind.
- Hold the ankle and gently bring in towards the body and tilt the pelvis back until a comfortable stretch is felt across the front of the thigh.

Awareness points
- Maintain a normal lumbar curve at all times.
- Avoid twisting the knee.

Alternatives
Side lying quad stretch

127

Exercise 14.6 Hip flexor stretch

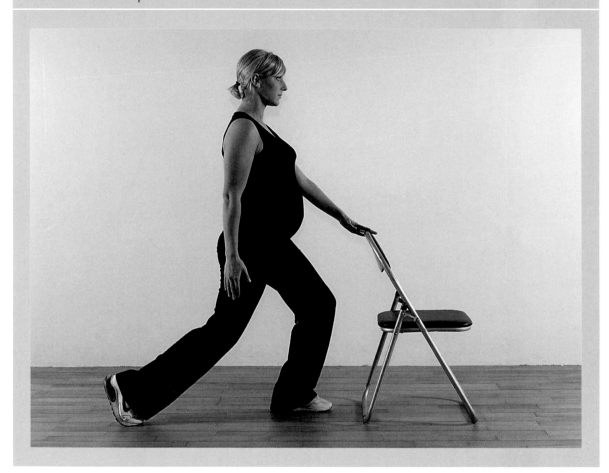

Major muscles used
Rectus femoris, hip flexors

Action
- Stand next to a stable support. Keep the spine in a neutral position.
- Take one foot back.
- Keeping the heel of the back foot lifted, bend both knees and tilt the pelvis back until a comfortable stretch is felt across the front of the hip.

Awareness points
- Maintain a normal lumbar curve at all times.
- Avoid twisting the knee.

Alternatives
Side lying quad stretch, kneeling hip flexor stretch, seated hip flexor stretch

Exercise 14.7 Calf stretch

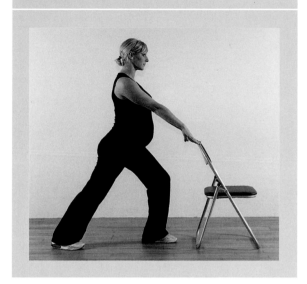

Major muscles used
Gastrocnemius and soleus

Action
- Stand next to a stable support. Keep the spine in a neutral position.
- Take one foot back and place the foot flat on the floor.
- Keeping the heel of the back foot flat and the back leg straight bend the front knee and lean forward until a comfortable stretch is felt in the calf of the back leg.

Awareness points
- Maintain a normal lumbar curve at all times.
- Avoid twisting the knee.
- Keep the body in a straight line from heel to head.

Alternatives
Seated calf stretch

Exercise 14.8 Adapted lower back stretch

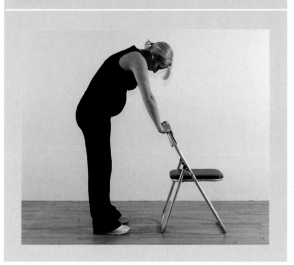

Major muscles used
Erector spinae

Action
- Stand next to a stable support.
- Hold the support and round the back into a curve.

Awareness points
Round from the lower back.

Alternatives
Seated lower back stretch

TA (TRANSVERSUS ABDOMINIS) CONTRACTION EXERCISES

Exercise 14.9 Kneeling abdominal hollow

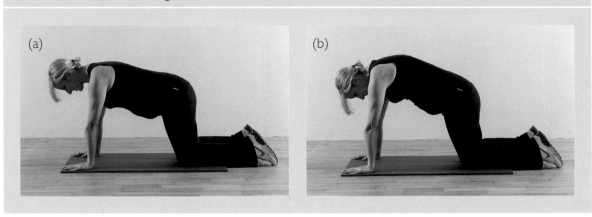

Start position

- Kneel on the floor with the shoulders directly above the hands and the hips directly above the knees.
- Keep the head facing down towards the floor to prevent undue stress on the cervical spine.
- Keep the knees shoulder width apart. Check that the spine is in the neutral position.

Action

- Consciously contract the transversus abdominis (TA).
- Breathe gently in and out while maintaining contraction.
- After a breath out and before breathing in again try to hollow the lower abdominals (imagine pulling the navel towards the spine).
- Hold this position for a few seconds or until you are not able while you continue to breathe normally.
- Repeat and try to maintain normal breathing throughout.

- Concentrate on keeping the starting position during the course of the exercise.

Progression

- Try to perform the action without contracting the rectus abdominis.
- Once comfortable with the above action, try to perform abdominal hollowing in a standing position.
- Try to contract the transversus abdominis without drawing in the lower abdominals. This is known as 'abdominal bracing'.

Exercise 14.10 Kneeling/All fours foot slide

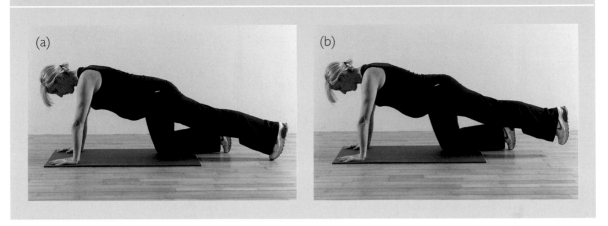

(a) (b)

Start position

- Kneel on the floor with the shoulders directly above the hands and the hips directly above the knees.
- Keep the head facing down towards the floor to prevent undue stress on the cervical spine.
- Keep the knees shoulder width apart. Check that the spine is in the neutral position.

Action

- Consciously contract the transversus abdominis.
- Breathe gently in and out while maintaining contraction.
- After a breath out and before breathing in again contract the lower abdominals as in 14.9a (imagine pulling the navel towards the spine).
- Hold this position and slowly slide the toe of one leg along the floor until the leg is extended (14.10a). Return to start and repeat with the other leg.
- Try to maintain normal breathing throughout.
- Concentrate on keeping the abdominals engaged during the course of the exercise.

Progression

- Try the all fours leg lift, starting as for the all fours foot slide.
- When leg is fully extended lift the foot a few inches off the floor as in 14.10b, lower, return to start position and repeat on other side.
- Ensure abdominals are engaged throughout and avoid allowing the spine to drop out of neutral position.

Adaptation

If pressure on the wrists makes this position uncomfortable, try placing the forearms on a low chair instead.

Exercise 14.11 Supine foot slide

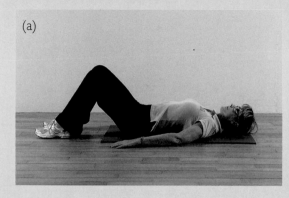

(a)

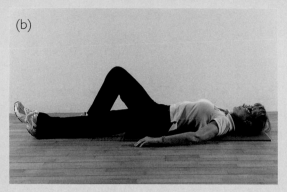

(b)

Start position

- Lie on your back with your feet flat on the floor and knees bent as far as is comfortably possible.
- Place one arm down by the side and the other under the lumbar spine to check the pressure on the hand throughout the exercise.
- Keep the knees shoulder width apart. Check that the spine is in the neutral position (14.11a).

Action

- Consciously contract the transversus abdominis.
- Breathe gently in and out.
- Slowly slide the foot outwards along the floor until the leg is fully extended (14.11b).
- Return to the start position and try to maintain normal breathing throughout.
- Concentrate on keeping the spine in the neutral position during the exercise so that the pressure on the hand does not change.

Progression

- Once comfortable with the above action, try increasing the speed of the movement slightly.
- If the above exercise can be performed without a change in pressure on the hand under the lumbar spine, try sliding both legs out and back at the same time.

Caution

Avoid supine positions after 16–18 weeks of pregnancy. Replace with the all fours foot slide (exercise 10, page 131).

Exercise 14.12 Supine pelvic tilts

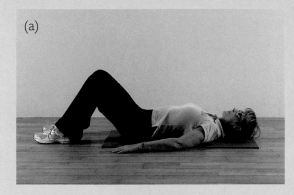
(a)

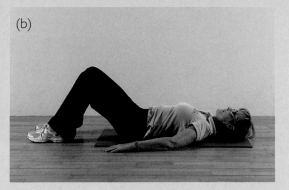
(b)

Start position

- Lie on your back with your feet flat on the floor and knees bent as far as is comfortably possible.
- Place the arms by the side.
- Keep the knees shoulder width apart. Check that the spine is in the neutral position (14.12a).

Action

- Consciously contract the transversus abdominis.
- Breathe gently in and out.
- Tilt the pelvis backwards so that the lower back is flat on the floor (14.12b).
- Return to the start position and try to maintain normal breathing throughout.

Progression

- Try the above exercise while lifting one foot slightly off the floor.
- As well as tilting the pelvis backwards, try and tilt the pelvis forwards so that the lumbar spine is arched more than normal.

Caution

Avoid supine positions after 16–18 weeks. Replace with all fours tilts or stability ball pelvic tilts (exercise 14.15, page 135).

Exercise 14.13 Stability ball sit

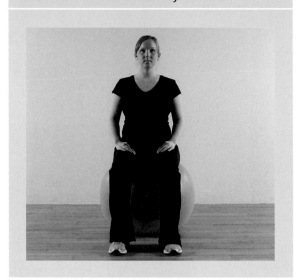

Exercise 14.14 Stability ball seated TA engagement

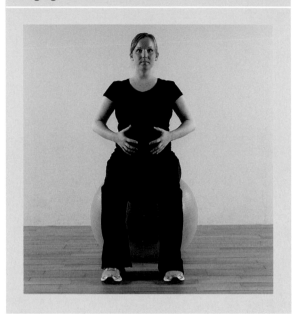

Start position
- Sit on the stability ball with feet flat on the floor and spine in an upright neutral position.
- Relax the shoulders down away from the ears.
- Widen the feet to increase stability.

Action
- Breathe gently in and out while holding this position.
- Avoid contracting the abdominals – focus on sitting tall.

Progression
Progress to stability ball TA engagement (exercise 14), with heel lifts and knee lifts only when upright posture can be maintained for up to 30 seconds.

Adaptation
Use a stability pad or disc on a chair to improve stability.

Start position
- Sit on the stability ball with feet flat on the floor and spine in an upright neutral position.
- Relax the shoulders down away from the ears.
- Widen the feet to increase stability.

Action
- Consciously contract the transversus abdominis.
- Breathe gently in and out.
- Hold for up to 20 seconds.

Progression
Stability ball seated pelvic tilts (exercise 15, page 135).

Adaptation
Use a stability pad or a disc on a chair to increase stability.

Exercise 14.15 Stability ball seated pelvic tilts

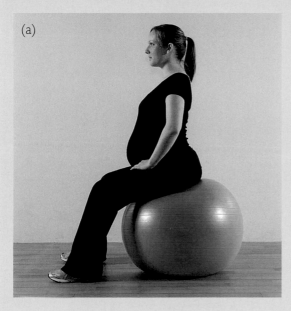

(a)

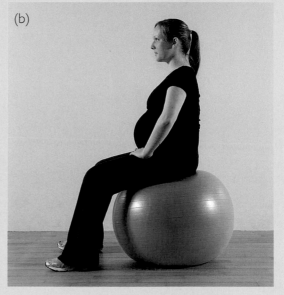

(b)

Start position

- Sit on the stability ball with feet flat on the floor and spine in an upright neutral position.
- Relax the shoulders down away from the ears.
- Widen the feet to increase stability.

Action

- Consciously contract the transversus abdominis.
- Breathe gently in and out.
- Gently tilt the pelvis forwards (14.15a) and backwards (14.15b) while maintaining upright posture.

Progression

Stability ball seated heel lifts and knee lifts (exercises 16 and 17, page 136).

Adaptation

Use a stability pad or a disc on a chair to increase stability.

Note!

Stability ball exercises should only be included if the client has been doing these for some time. Consider using a stability pad or disc on a chair for newcomers to exercise.

Exercise 14.16 Stability ball seated heel lifts

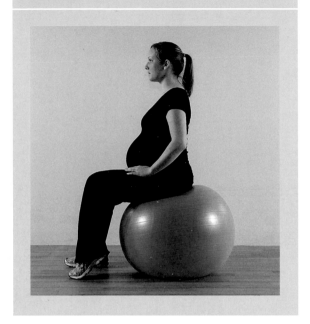

Exercise 14.17 Stability ball seated knee lifts

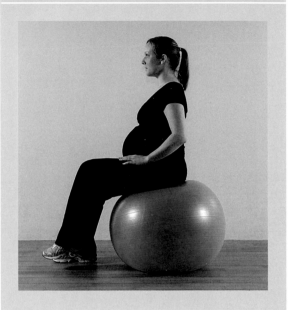

Start position

- Sit on the stability ball with feet flat on the floor and spine in an upright neutral position.
- Relax the shoulders down away from the ears.
- Widen the feet to increase stability.

Action

- Consciously contract the transversus abdominis.
- Breathe gently in and out.
- Gently lift one heel off the floor and hold.
- Replace and repeat on the other side.

Progression

Knee lifts (exercise 17).

Adaptation

Use a stability pad or a disc on a chair to increase stability.

Start position

- Sit on the stability ball with feet flat on the floor and spine in an upright neutral position.
- Relax the shoulders down away from the ears.
- Widen the feet to increase stability.

Action

- Consciously contract the transversus abdominis.
- Breathe gently in and out.
- Gently lift one knee and hold.
- Replace and repeat on the other side.

Adaptation

Use a stability pad or a disc on a chair to increase stability.

SHOULDER STABILISATION EXERCISES

With all band exercises, the tension on the band can be increased or decreased to suit the individual. The band should be attached to a fixed securing point.

Exercise 14.18 The Dumb Waiter

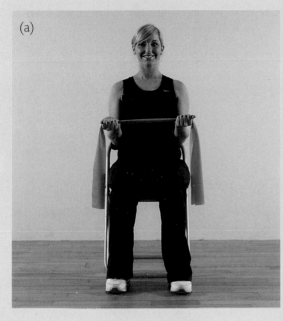
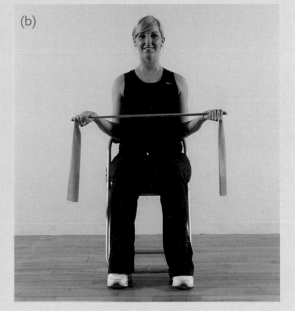

(a)

(b)

Start position
- Sit in a chair slightly towards the front of the seat with the feet flat on the floor.
- Keep the spine in a neutral position with the head looking forward.
- Bend the elbows to a right angle keeping them close to the body and hold the band about shoulder width apart with palms facing up.

Action
- Consciously contract the transversus abdominis.
- Keep the elbows close to the body and take the hands out as wide as is comfortable.

- Keep the shoulders down and the chest lifted throughout the exercise.

Progression
- Have the hands closer together on the band at the start.
- Use a higher resistance band.

Adaptation
Perform the move without a band.

137

Exercise 14.19 Upper back strengthener

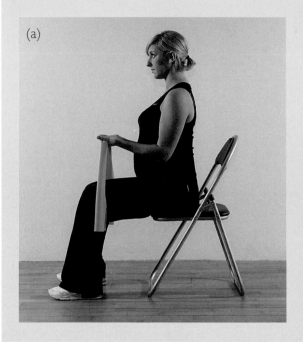

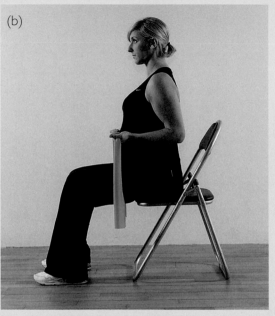

Start position
- Sit in a chair slightly towards the front of the seat with the feet flat on the floor.
- Keep the spine in a neutral position with the head looking forward.
- Bend the elbows to a right angle keeping them close to the body and hold the band about 6–8 inches apart with palms facing up.

Action
- Consciously contract the transversus abdominis.
- Take the hands apart increasing tension on the band.
- Pull the elbows back as far as is comfortable while maintaining the tension on the band.
- Release back to start position.

- Keep the shoulders down and the chest lifted throughout the exercise.

Progression
- Have the hands closer together on the band at the start.
- Use a higher resistance band.

Adaptation
Perform the move without a band.

Exercise 14.20 Seated back extension (alternative to the back extension machine)

Start position

- Sit in a chair slightly towards the front of the seat with the feet flat on the floor.
- Keep the spine in a neutral position with the head looking forward and lean forwards.

Action

- Place the band securely under the feet and hold it under tension about 8 inches from the floor.
- Keeping the arms straight sit upright pivoting from the hip.

Exercise 14.21 Internal rotation

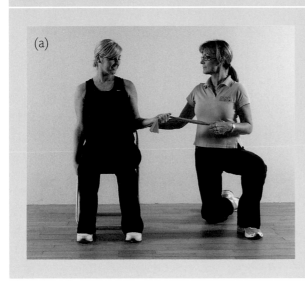

(a)

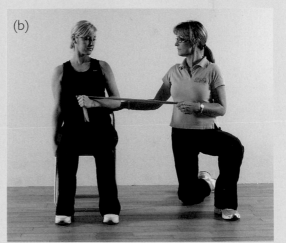

(b)

Start position

- Secure the band at waist level.
- Stand with the feet shoulder width apart.
- Sit on a chair side-on to the direction of the resistance band, take hold of the band with the nearest arm to the securing point.
- Keep the upper arm tucked into the side with the lower arm parallel to the floor and away from the body as in the start position (14.21a).
- Take a position so that the band is slightly on stretch.

- Check that the spine is in the neutral position.

Action

- Consciously contract the transversus abdominis.
- With the upper arm kept tight to the body, rotate so that the lower arm comes towards the body (end position 14.21b).
- Gently return to the starting point.
- Maintain normal breathing throughout.

Exercise 14.22 External rotation

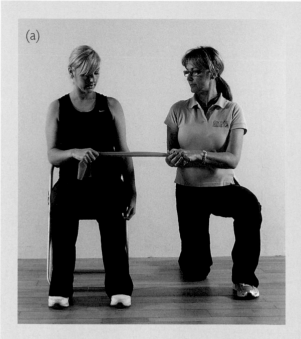

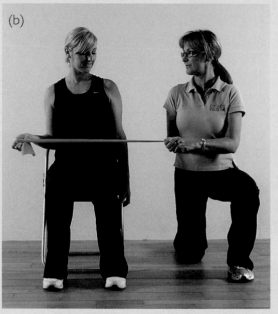

Start position

- Secure the band at waist level.
- Sit on a chair with the feet shoulder width apart.
- Facing side-on to the direction of the resistance band, take hold of the band with the farthest arm to the securing point.
- Keep the upper arm tucked into the side with the lower arm parallel to the floor and across the body as in the start position (14.22a).
- Take a position so that the band is slightly on stretch.
- Check that the spine is in the neutral position.

Action

- Consciously contract the transversus abdominis.
- With the upper arm kept tight to the body, rotate so that the lower arm moves away from the body (end position 14.22b).
- Gently return to the starting point.
- Maintain normal breathing throughout.

Exercise 14.23 Shoulder abduction

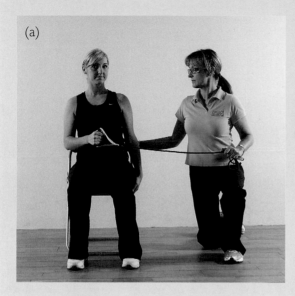
(a)

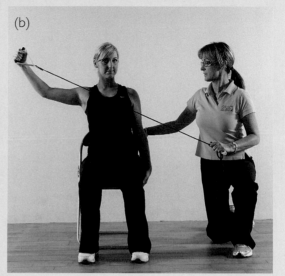
(b)

Start position

- Secure the band low to the ground.
- Sit on a chair with the feet shoulder width apart.
- Facing side-on to the direction of the resistance band, take hold of the handle.
- The arm should be across the body as in the start position (14.23a).
- Take a position so that the band is slightly on stretch.
- Check that the spine is in the neutral position.

Action

- Consciously contract the transversus abdominis.
- With the arm kept almost straight (slight elbow bend) bring the arm across the body to the end position (14.23b).
- Gently return to the starting point.
- Maintain normal breathing throughout.

Exercise 14.24 Shoulder adduction

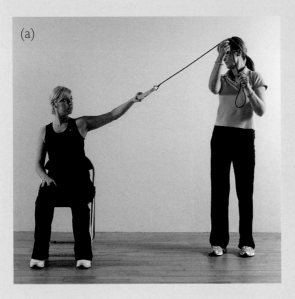

(a)

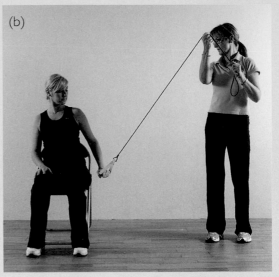

(b)

Start position

- Secure the band above head height.
- Sit on a chair with the feet shoulder width apart.
- Facing side-on to the direction of the resistance band, take hold of the handle.
- The arm should be out to the side of the body as in the start position (14.24a).
- Take a position so that the band is slightly on stretch.
- Check that the spine is in the neutral position.

Action

- Consciously contract the transversus abdominis.
- With the arm kept almost straight (slight elbow bend) bring the arm down alongside the body to the end position (14.24b).
- Gently return to the starting point.
- Maintain normal breathing throughout.

HIP STABILISATION EXERCISES

With all band exercises, the tension on the band can be increased or decreased to suit the individual. The band should be attached to a fixed securing point.

Exercise 14.25 Hip abduction

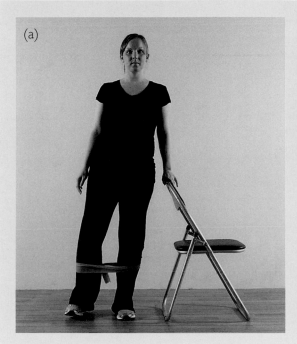
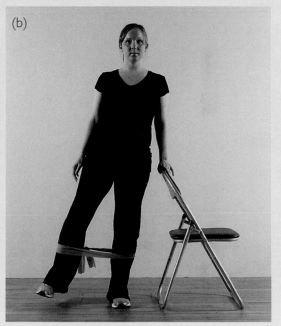

Start position
- Secure the band around the mid calf.
- Stand with the feet hip width apart (14.25a).
- Ensure there is slight tension on the band.
- Check that the spine is in the neutral position.

Action
- Consciously contract the transversus abdominis.
- With the leg kept almost straight, take the leg out to the side to the end position (14.25b).
- Try not to let the hips rotate at all.
- Gently return to the starting point.
- Maintain normal breathing throughout.

Alternative
Seated band abduction

Exercise 14.26 Seated band abduction

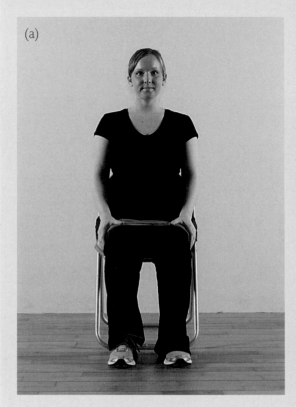
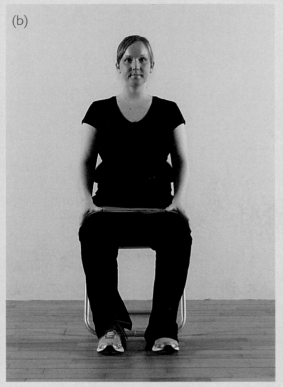

(a)

(b)

Start position

- Sit in a stable chair with the bottom towards the front of the seat and feet hip width apart.
- Wrap the band round the thighs keeping it flat. Hold the ends securely.

Action

- Consciously contract the transversus abdominis.
- Take the legs out to the sides then return to start position.

Exercise 14.27 Hip adduction

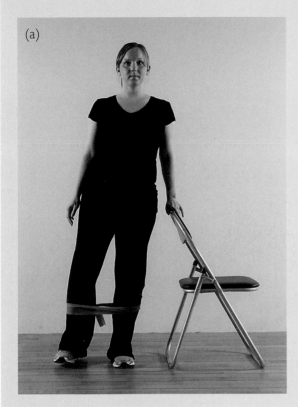
(a)

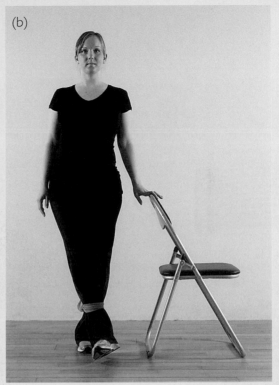
(b)

Start position

- Secure the band around the mid calf.
- Stand with the feet hip width apart (14.27a).
- Ensure there is slight tension in the band.
- Check that the spine is in the neutral position.

Action

- Consciously contract the transversus abdominis.
- Shift the weight onto the inside leg.
- With the attached leg kept almost straight, bring the leg slightly across the body to the end position (14.27b).
- Try not to let the hips rotate at all.
- Gently return to the starting point.
- Maintain normal breathing throughout.

Alternative

Circle squeeze

Exercise 14.28 Circle squeeze

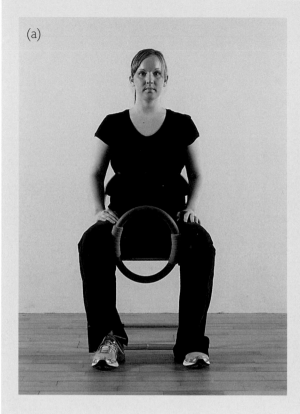

(a)

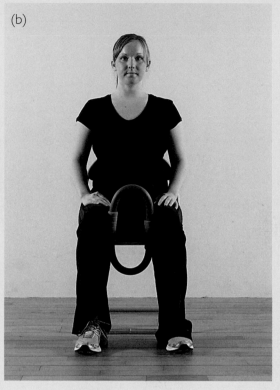

(b)

Start position

- Sit in a stable chair with the bottom towards the front of the seat and feet hip width apart.
- Place a circle between the knees.

Action

- Consciously contract the transversus abdominis.
- Squeeze the knees towards each other then release.

Exercise 14.29 Hip extension

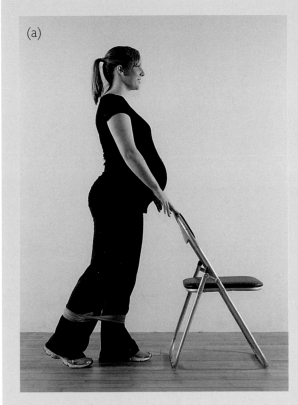
(a)

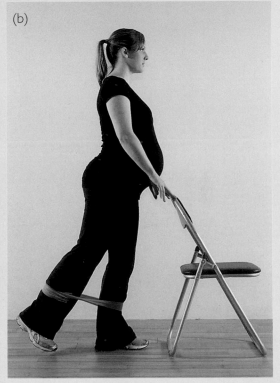
(b)

Start position

- Secure the band around the lower legs.
- Stand with the feet close together.
- Face the direction of support.
- Take a position so that the band is slightly on stretch.
- Check that the spine is in the neutral position (14.29a).

Action

- Consciously contract the transversus abdominis.
- Shift the weight onto the front leg.
- With the front leg kept almost straight, take the back leg directly backwards (14.29b).
- Try not to let the hips rotate at all.
- Gently return to the starting point.
- Maintain normal breathing throughout.
- Repeat for the other side.

Exercise 14.30 Hip flexion

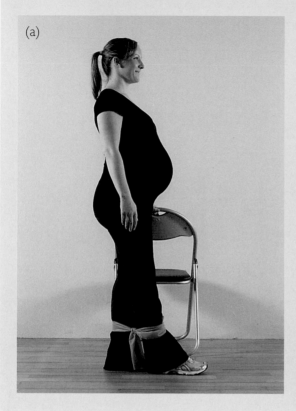

(a)

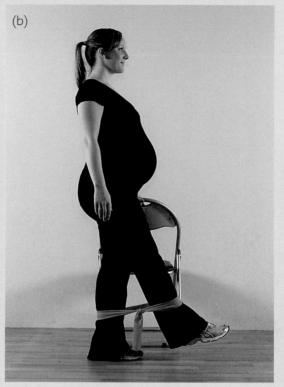

(b)

Start position

- Secure the band around the mid calf.
- Stand with the feet close together (14.30a).
- Ensure there is slight tension in the band.
- Check that the spine is in the neutral position.

Action

- Consciously contract the transversus abdominis.
- Shift the weight onto the inside leg.
- With the outside leg kept almost straight, take the leg directly forwards (14.30b).
- Try not to let the hips rotate at all.
- Gently return to the starting point.
- Maintain normal breathing throughout.

MOBILISATION EXERCISES

Exercise 14.31 Chest press (free weights)

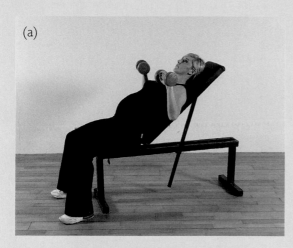

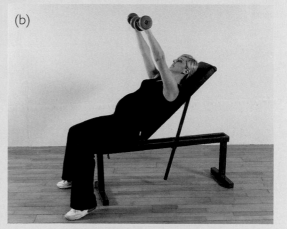

Major muscles used

Pectoralis major

Supporting muscles used

Anterior deltoid, tricep, serratus anterior

Start position

- Lie on the bench and make sure the feet are placed firmly on the ground and that the upper arms are extended away from the body (start position 14.31a).
- The palms should be facing forwards and the hands should be directly above the elbows.
- Grip the weights so that they are also parallel to the floor.

Action

- Raise the weights in an arcing motion keeping them in line with the chest until the arms are fully extended (end position 14.31b).
- Lower the arms under control back to the start position.

Awareness points

- Keep the hands directly above the elbows at all times and make sure that the wrists remain firm.
- Lower the weights under control until the elbows are below the shoulders.
- Maintain a normal lumbar curve at all times.

Alternatives

Machine chest press, chest flye, pec dec, box press-up, wall press-up.

Caution

Avoid lying on the back after 16–18 weeks.

Exercise 14.32 Chest press (machine)

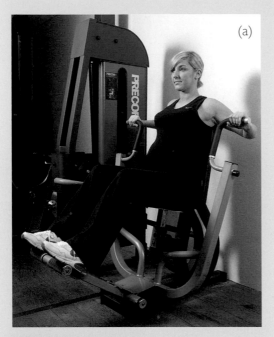

(a)

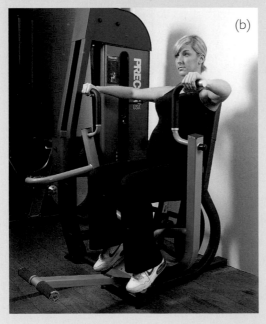

(b)

Major muscles used
Pectoralis major

Supporting muscles used
Anterior deltoid, triceps, serratus anterior

Start position
- Make sure the seat is at the height where the handles are about chest level.
- Take an overhand grip.
- The upper arms should be level with the body and not extended behind it (14.32a).

Action
- Fully extend the arms keeping the wrists firm and in a straight line with the forearm (end position 14.32b).
- Return to the start position under control.

Awareness points
- Maintain a normal lumbar curve at all times.
- Do not allow the hands to go out of peripheral vision at any time by taking the upper arms behind the line of the body.

Alternatives
Free-weight chest press, chest flye, pec dec, press-ups (box or wall).

Caution
May be uncomfortable for the breasts in later stages of pregnancy.

Exercise 14.33 Single arm row (free weights)

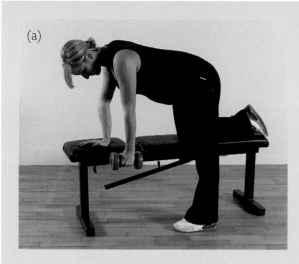

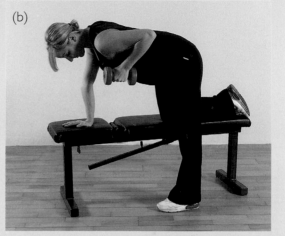

Major muscles used
Latissimus dorsi

Supporting muscles used
Biceps brachialis, posterior deltoid

Start position
- Adopt a kneeling position on one leg on a bench so that the hip joint of that leg is approximately 90 degrees and the supporting hand is directly below the shoulder.
- Place the supporting leg on the ground slightly away from the bench but at the level of the hip joint.
- Fully extend the arm down holding the weight with the palm turned inwards (14.33a).

Action
- Draw the weight toward the upper body until the upper arm is parallel with the floor (end position 14.33b).
- Return the weight to the start position under control.

Awareness points
- Keep the head facing down to maintain neutral cervical spine.
- Maintain a normal lumbar curve at all times.

Alternatives
Lat pull down, seated row

Exercise 14.34 Lat pull down (machine)

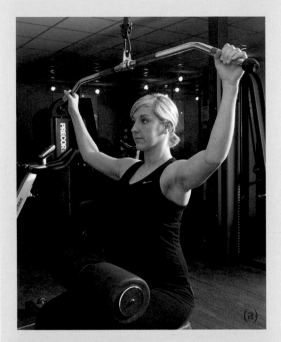

(a)

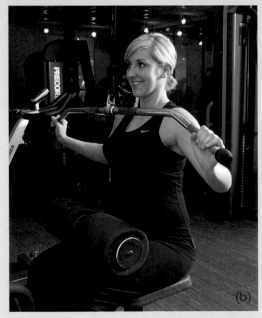

(b)

Major muscles used
Latissimus dorsi

Supporting muscles used
Biceps brachialis, posterior deltoid

Start position
- With the feet firmly on the floor and spine in neutral, take a seat.
- Adjust the seat height so that the arms are almost at full extension when gripping the handles on the bar.
- Place the knees under the restraint pad if fitted.
- Reach up and grasp the bar handles firmly with both hands (14.34a).

Action
- Draw the bar vertically down in front of the body until the bar is roughly in line with the chin (end position 14.34b).
- Return to the start position under control.

Awareness points
- Keep the head facing forwards to maintain neutral cervical spine.
- Maintain a normal lumbar curve at all times.
- Only draw the bar to chin level to avoid undue strain on the rotator cuff muscles by preventing internal rotation.
- Draw the bar to the front of the body to avoid stress on the shoulder joints.

Alternatives
Seated row, single-arm row

Caution
Your bump may get in the way of the machine in later stages of pregnancy.

Exercise 14.35 Shoulder press (free weights)

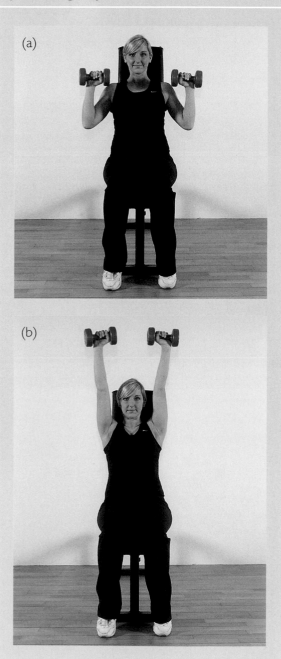

(a)

(b)

Major muscles used
Deltoids (anterior and posterior)

Supporting muscles used
Triceps

Start position
- With the feet shoulder width apart and spine in neutral position, make sure that the upper arms are slightly below parallel position.
- The hands should be directly above the elbow joint.
- The palms should be facing forwards and the hands should be in peripheral vision (14.35a).

Action
- Raise the weights in an arcing motion keeping them in peripheral vision at all times until the arms are fully extended (end position 14.35b).
- Return to the start position under control.

Awareness points
- Both hands should remain within peripheral vision at all times in order to protect the shoulder joint.
- Maintain a normal lumbar curve at all times.

Alternatives
Machine shoulder press, lateral raise, upright row

Exercise 14.36 Lateral raise (free weights)

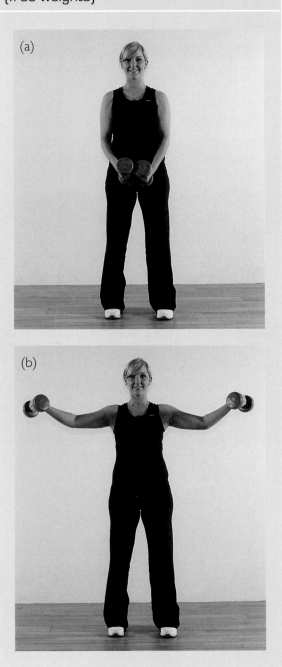

(a)

(b)

Major muscles used
Deltoids (anterior and posterior)

Supporting muscles used
Trapezius (upper fibres during shoulder elevation)

Start position
- The feet should be shoulder width apart and spine in neutral position.
- Arms should hang by the sides with a slight bend at the elbow joint so that the weight is slightly forward of the hip joint.
- The palms should be facing inwards (14.36a).

Action
- Raise the weights in an abduction motion keeping them in line slightly forward of the hip joint until the arms are parallel to the floor (end position 14.36b).
- Return to the start position under control.

Awareness points
- Both hands should remain within peripheral vision at all times.
- Maintain a normal lumbar curve at all times.
- Stop when the arms are parallel to the floor to avoid impingement at the acromioclavicular joint.

Alternatives
Shoulder press, upright row

Exercise **14.37** Shoulder press (machine)

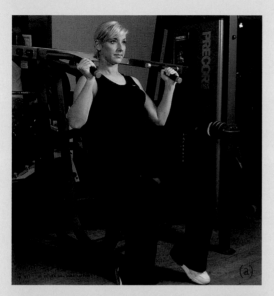

(a)

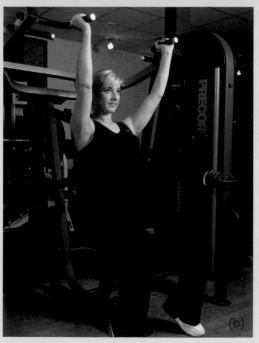

(b)

Major muscles used
Deltoids (anterior and posterior)

Supporting muscles used
Triceps

Start position
* Sit on the seat and keep the feet firmly on the ground and the spine in neutral position.
* Adjust the seat height until the upper arms are slightly below parallel position when holding the handles (14.37a).

Action
* Raise the arms until they are fully extended (end position 14.37b).
* Return to the start position under control.

Awareness points
* Both hands should remain within peripheral vision at all times.
* Maintain a normal lumbar curve at all times.

Alternatives
Free-weight shoulder press, lateral raise, upright row

Exercise 14.38 Triceps extension (free weights)

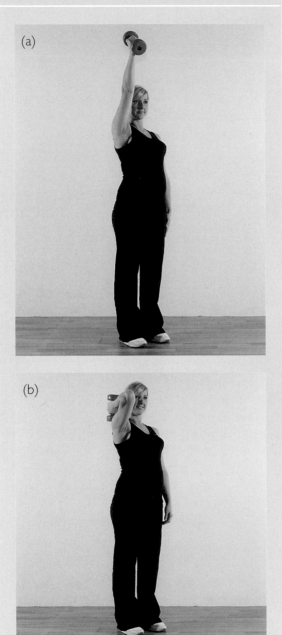

(a)

(b)

Major muscles used
Triceps

Supporting muscles used
Anconeus

Start position
- The feet should be shoulder width apart and the spine in neutral position.
- Grasping the weight, the upper arm is extended directly above the head with a 90 degree bend at the elbow.
- The palm should be facing inwards (14.38a).

Action
- Extend the arm so that the hand is directly above the shoulder joint (end position 14.38b).
- Return to the start position under control.

Awareness points
- Maintain a normal lumbar curve at all times.
- Make sure that the weight remains to the side of the head at all times.

Alternatives
Triceps push, triceps kick-back, narrow-arm press-up

Exercise 14.39 Triceps kick-back (free weights)

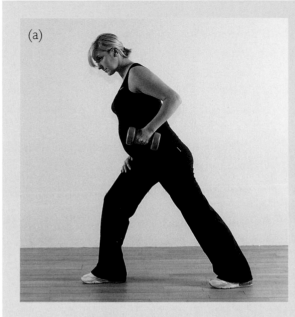
(a)

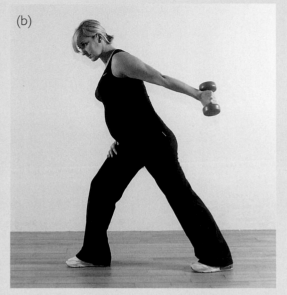
(b)

Major muscles used
Triceps

Supporting muscles used
Anconeus

Start position
- Adopt a split stance position with the front leg bent and the back leg straight.
- Place the hand on the thigh of the front leg.
- Lean into the front knee and ensure the body is in a straight line from head to back heel.

Action
- Extend the lower arm backwards until it is parallel with the floor (end position 14.39b).
- Return to the start position under control.

Awareness points
- Keep the head facing down to maintain neutral cervical spine.
- Maintain a normal lumbar curve at all times.

Alternatives
Triceps push, triceps extension, narrow-arm press-up

Exercise 14.40 Triceps push (machine)

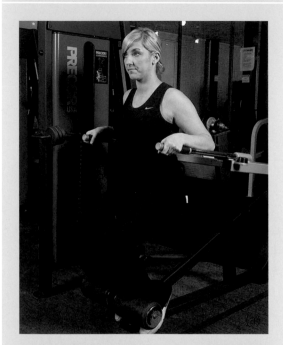

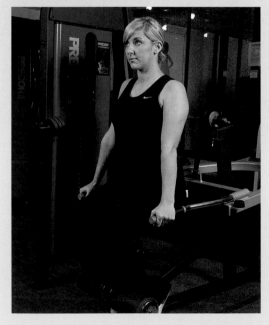

Major muscles used
Triceps

Supporting muscles used
Anconeus

Start position
- Sit firmly on the seat and keep the feet firmly on the ground and the spine in a neutral position.
- Adjust the seat height so that the forearms are about parallel to the floor (14.40a).

Action
- Extend the lower arm so that the arms are both fully straight (end position 14.40b).
- Return to the start position under control.

Awareness points
Maintain a normal lumbar curve at all times.

Alternatives
Triceps extension, triceps kick-back, narrow-arm press-up

Exercise 14.41 Biceps curl (free weights)

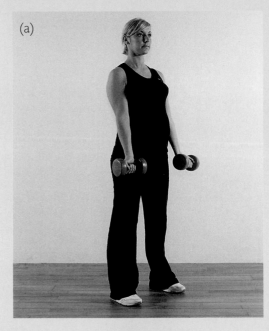

(a)

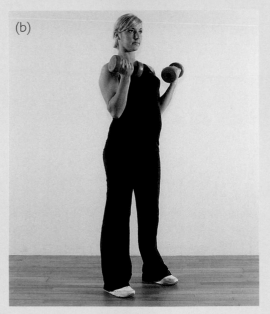

(b)

Major muscles used
Biceps brachii

Supporting muscles used
Biceps brachialis, brachioradialis

Start position
- The feet should be shoulder width apart and the spine in a neutral position.
- The arms should hang by the sides with the palms facing forwards (this is called the anatomical position) as in 14.41a.

Action
- Raise the weights in a line towards, but clear of, the face, as shown (end position 14.41b).
- Return to the start position under control.

Awareness points
- Maintain a normal lumbar curve at all times.
- Make sure that the weights do not strike the face and lower to full extension of the elbow joint.

Alternatives
Biceps curl machine

HIP MOBILISATION EXERCISES

Exercise 14.42 Squat (free weights)

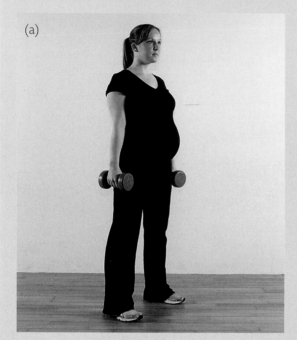

(a)

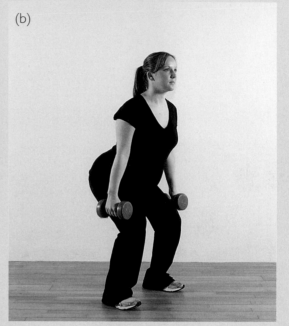

(b)

Major muscles used

Quadriceps, hamstrings, gluteus maximus, erector spinae

Supporting muscles used

Some of the muscles above work as synergists depending on the angle of the torso.

Start position

*   The feet should be shoulder width apart and the spine in a neutral position.
*   The arms should hang by the sides with the palms facing inwards and grasping the weights (if used) firmly (14.42a).

Action

*   Bend the hip joint and knee joint as in a sitting motion to a point that feels comfortable (end position 14.42b).
*   Return to the start position, under control.

Awareness points

*   Maintain a normal lumbar curve at all times.
*   The head should drop and raise in a vertical line so that the body does not tilt forward.
*   Encourage the maximum range of motion.

Alternatives

Squat machine

Exercise 14.43 Lunge (free weights)

(a)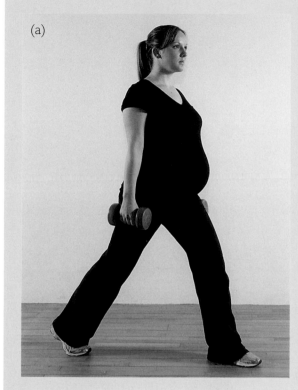

(b)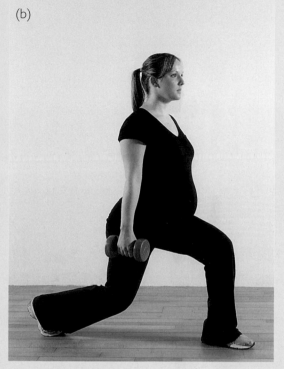

Major muscles used
Quadriceps, hamstrings, gluteus maximus, erector spinae

Supporting muscles used
Some of the muscles above work as synergists if the torso is angled forwards.

Start position
- The feet should be one in front of the other and the spine in a neutral position.
- The arms should hang by the sides with the palms facing inwards and grasping the weights (if used) firmly (14.43a).

Action
- Take a small step forward with one leg and lower the back leg as if trying to put the knee on the floor. Keep the body in an upright position (end position 14.43b).
- Return to the start position under control.
- Repeat on the other side.

Awareness points
- Maintain a normal lumbar curve at all times.
- Try not to let the knee of the front foot go beyond the toes.

Exercise 14.44 Calf Raise

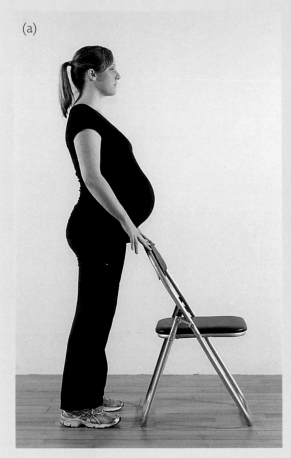

(a)

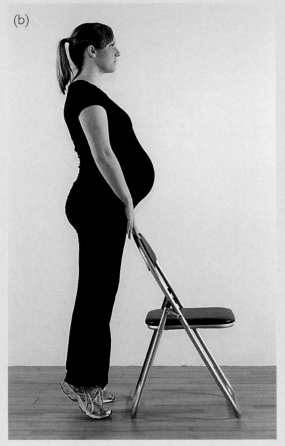

(b)

Major muscles used

Gastrocnemius and soleus

Supporting muscles used

Soleus

Start position

- Stand close to a stable form of support with the feet hip width or further apart.

Action

- Raise up onto the toes keeping the spine neutral.
- Lower under control back to the start position.

Exercise **14.45** Leg extension (machine)

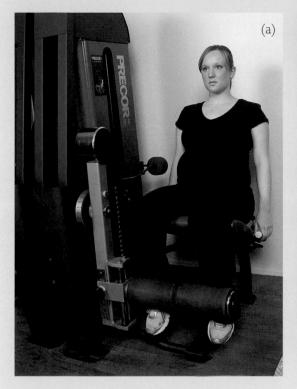

(a)

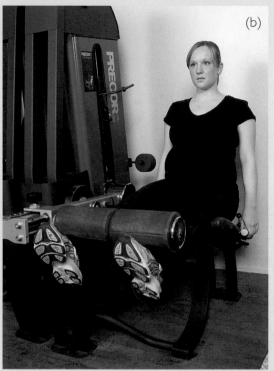

(b)

Major muscles used
Quadriceps

Supporting muscles used
None used as isolates the quadriceps

Start position
- Sit on the machine and place the roller pads just above the ankle joint.
- Use the machine seat setting to move the seat so that the knee joint is just at the edge of the seat.
- Start with the knees flexed as far as comfortably possible (14.45a).

Action
- Extend the knees to full range of motion (end position 14.45b).
- Return to the start position under control.

Awareness points
- Maintain a normal lumbar curve at all times.
- Keep the knees and the toes pointing directly upwards at all times.
- Ensure that full extension is achieved.

Alternatives
Squats, leg press, lunges

Exercise 14.46 Seated leg curl (machine)

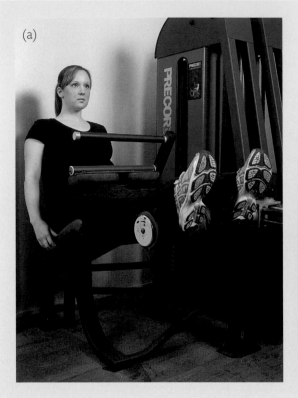

(a)

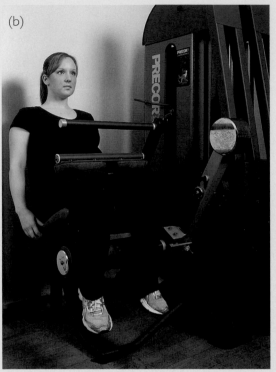

(b)

Major muscles used
Hamstrings

Supporting muscles used
Calf

Start position
- Sit on the machine and place the roller pads just above the calcaneus or heel bone.
- Use the machine seat setting to move the seat so that the knee joint is just at the edge of the seat.
- Start with the knees extended as far as comfortably possible (14.46a).

Action
- Flex the knees to full range of motion (end position 14.46b).
- Return to the start position under control.

Awareness points
- Maintain a normal lumbar curve at all times.
- Keep the knees and the toes pointing directly upwards at all times.

Alternatives
Squats, leg press, lunges

RELAXATION DURING PREGNANCY

15

Relaxation is acknowledged as an important part of an antenatal or postnatal session and this component of a session can last for a minute or two or longer. It is a useful technique for the mother to learn as it can be very refreshing during periods of reduced or interrupted sleep.

The actual relaxation can involve controlled breathing, visualisation, passive or active progressive muscular relaxation or a method such as the Mitchell Method which is particularly suited to pregnancy. Visit http://www.acpwh.org.uk/docs/RelaxationLeaflet.pdf to download a leaflet on the Mitchell Method.

The position adopted for relaxation will need to be adapted after 16–18 weeks to avoid supine hypotensive syndrome and the following positions are recommended.

SIDE LYING 'RECOVERY' POSITION

Lie on the side and position the top leg so that the knee is bent and in front of the body at an angle that feels comfortable (see figure 15.1). Position the arms where comfortable, the bottom arm may be behind the body and the top arm in front. For comfort, a pillow or cushion under the head and breasts, and between the top knee and ankle,

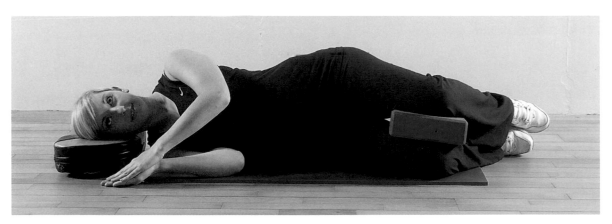

Figure 15.1 Side lying 'recovery' position

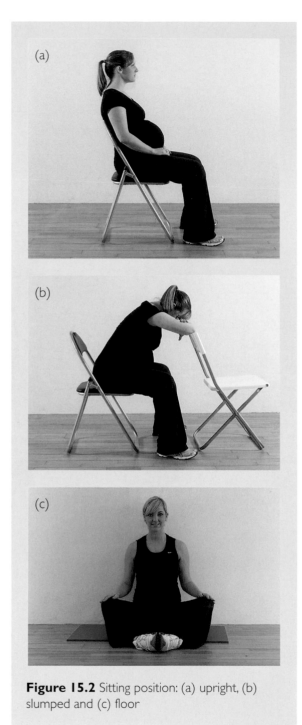

Figure 15.2 Sitting position: (a) upright, (b) slumped and (c) floor

could be used. Allow time to adjust the position to the most comfortable.

SITTING POSITION 1: UPRIGHT

Choose a comfortable chair with arms if available, and of a height that allows both feet to be flat on the floor. Use cushions or back support in the lumbar region if needed.

SITTING POSITION 2: SLUMPED

Sit in a chair with the feet flat on the floor and lean forward resting the head on the arms or a cushion on a table or other stable surface.

SITTING POSITION 3: FLOOR

Sit with the back against a wall or other solid upright surface. Position the legs as comfortable, the knees can be straight out or bent, crossed or not. Position cushions under the knees, in the lumbar region, or under the bottom as preferred.

When getting down to the floor or back up again ensure a safe method is used to minimise the risk of falling or of straining the abdominal muscles. Use a chair or wall for support and lower onto one knee then bring the other knee alongside. Gently move onto all fours then sit sideways onto one hip before either moving into a seated position against a wall or, if moving into a side lying position, gently slide the arm out along the floor until the body is safely on the floor. Reverse the process to get back up again; from side lying push the body up into a sitting position then move onto the hands and knees. Bring one leg up in front so the knee is bent and the foot flat on the floor. Use the thigh as a lever to push the body up into an upright position.

Always include a few revitalising moves after any period of relaxation to shake off any drowsiness.

POSTNATAL ACTIVITY

16

EXERCISES FOR THE IMMEDIATE POSTNATAL PERIOD

During the immediate postnatal period the new mother is likely to be experiencing tiredness, emotional mood swings and anxiety so exercise is probably the last thing on her mind. 'Normal' exercise or activity should not be resumed until after the six-week check-up confirms that it is all right to do so as everything is back to normal in terms of body physiology. However, some gentle activity in the immediate postnatal period may help with fatigue and mood and provide a welcome time-out. Therefore, provided the new mother is feeling up to it, the following exercise guidelines are recommended.

CARDIOVASCULAR

- Walking is the best activity during the immediate postnatal period and a daily gentle to brisk walk should be encouraged.
- Swimming can be resumed once the lochia discharge has ceased. Avoid breaststroke leg motion initially if pelvic girdle pain is present.
- Gentle stationary cycling is a suitable low impact activity for this time period, provided that the pelvic and genital regions have recovered!

MUSCULAR STRENGTH AND ENDURANCE

- Lifting and carrying the new baby will probably be enough at this stage but squats and calf raises will help with circulation and strength.
- Stair climbing is good for the legs and should be actively encouraged.

BREASTFEEDING

Advise new mothers to maintain correct posture when breastfeeding to avoid postural imbalances (see figure 16.1). A kyphotic, round shouldered posture is common when breastfeeding so correct positioning of the baby using cushions or pillows should be practised prior to delivery and maintained during the feeding period.

CORE EXERCISES

It is essential that strengthening around the core (trunk) area is carried out throughout the pregnancy and afterwards as the strain on this area due to the increased load of the baby is immense. Abdominal and back strengthening exercises should be incorporated into all resistance training sessions, and it is likely that the new mother will have been give some gentle abdominal rehabilitation exercises by the obstetric physiotherapist or midwife shortly after birth and these should be encouraged. These usually consist of crook-lying head raises, small oblique movements, transversus abdominis engagement and the all-important pelvic floor contractions.

DIASTASIS RECTI

The other concern before doing any physical activity is related to the separation of the rectus abdominis muscle (or more accurately the linea

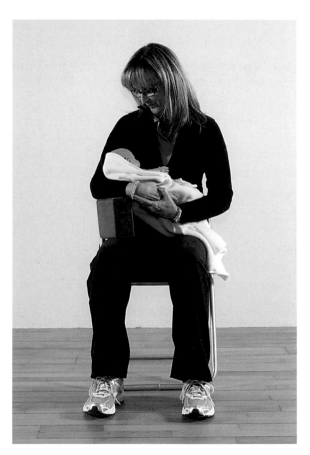

Figure 16.1 Correct feeding posture

alba). It is common that the rectus abdominis can separate by as much as 2cm (two–three finger gap) following delivery of the baby. It is important therefore that time is given to allow the muscle to return to its normal position. This normally takes a few weeks or even longer, so it is important to avoid certain exercises such as abdominal or oblique curls and sit-ups in this time period. If the separation is still extreme after the six-week check, any form of spinal flexion exercise should be omitted until the separation is less than two fingers' width.

It is relatively easy for mothers to check their own rectus abdominis to see if it is re-aligned and that the linea alba has healed. The check for diastasis recti (or 'rec check') can be done as follows:

- Lie on your back with knees bent and feet flat on the floor.
- Slide a hand under the lower back to check the lumbar curve. The hand should fit snugly.
- Raise the head and shoulders slightly off the floor (get someone to help if necessary) as this will cause the rectus abdominis to contract.
- Run the fingers across the abdomen above and below the belly button as in figure 16.2 (with light pressure only).
- Make sure you keep breathing throughout.

If the gap in the rectus abdominis is less than 3cm (about two fingers wide), this is an indication that the linea alba has fully healed and that the rectus has re-aligned. If the gap is wider than this, it is recommended that certain abdominal exercises, such as abdominal or oblique curls and sit-ups are **not** done as it could cause abdominal doming (which is a bulge in the abdominal wall).

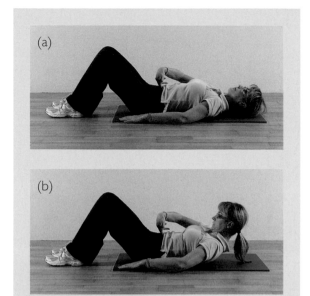

Figure 16.2 Checking the rectus abdominis: (a) start, (b) finish

This is also the case with a caesarean section, which is a surgical procedure that opens the abdomen and lower segment of the uterus to deliver a baby that cannot be born through the vagina. It is important to understand that if a mother has had a caesarean section birth, abdominal exercises should not be done until the rectus abdominis has re-aligned and the wound is fully healed. This can take as long as 12 weeks to heal and even then, exercises should be done carefully and with slow progression.

PELVIC FLOOR

The pelvic floor muscles become particularly weak during pregnancy due to the weight of the growing baby and can be stretched during delivery, so they need particular attention as they are responsible for bladder, uterus and rectum control.

The pelvic floor muscles can be strengthened using exercises known as 'Kegel' exercises. These exercises can be done by slowly and strongly squeezing the muscles that you use to stop the flow of urine or to avoid breaking wind. Hold this contraction for up to 10 seconds, then release slowly. To train the fast-twitch fibres, contract the area quickly, hold then release slowly. Do both fast and slow contractions 10–20 times in a row at least three times a day. This is not just a postnatal procedure but one that should be done during pregnancy and throughout life.

If an 'episiotomy' (a surgical procedure where an incision is made in the area between the anus and the vagina to widen the exit route for the baby) has been carried out, this can take about 10–15 days to heal and about six weeks for the stitches to dissolve. Pelvic floor exercises may help to speed up the healing process so these should be encouraged as long as they do not cause pain or discomfort.

For more information we recommend *The Complete Guide to Postnatal Fitness* by Judy DiFiore when working with post natal women.

APPENDIX 1 MOVEMENT DEFINITIONS

Term	Explanation	Picture
Flexion	The term flexion ('flex' meaning to bend) is used when the angle between the moving bones gets smaller. In the example shown the torso is bent forward (forward flexion of the spine or trunk).	
Extension	This is where the joint angle gets larger. An example of this could be a straight leg movement in a backwards direction as in a hip extension exercise. The example shown is where the torso is bent backward from a flexed position. This is known as extension of the spine or trunk.	
Lateral flexion or lateral extension	This refers to bending to the side as with the neck or spine. This can be seen in the example and is known as lateral flexion or extension of the spine or trunk.	

Rotation	This term is used to describe a bone revolving around its own axis. An example is rotation at the ulna-radius joint when turning the palm face down from a face-up position. Another example is shown where the head rotates from side to side, as if saying no.	
Abduction	Abduction describes a movement away from the midline of the body as shown. An example of this would be in a lateral shoulder raise where the upper arm moves away from the body (abduction of the humerus).	
Adduction	This is a term used to describe a movement toward the midline of the body as shown. An example of this would be the lat pull down as the upper arm would adduct (adduction of the humerus).	
Medial rotation	This describes any limb that rotates inward towards the body. The example shows the upper arm (humerus) rotating inward. This is known as a rotator cuff exercise.	
Lateral rotation	This describes any limb that rotates outwards away from the body. An example of this can be seen when the upper arm (humerus) rotates outward. This is also a rotator cuff exercise.	

Elevation	This term describes an upward movement of a part of the body such as lifting the shoulders up in a 'shoulder shrug' exercise.	
Depression	This term describes a downward movement of a part of the body such as the shoulders going down from an elevated position.	
Pronation	This term can be used to describe the palm or the sole of the foot being turned down.	
Supination	This term can be used to describe the palm or the sole of the foot being turned up.	
Inversion	The example shows the sole of the foot turned inwards.	

Eversion	The example shows the sole of the foot turned out.	
Plantar flexion	This term refers to bending the foot at the ankle joint so that the foot is pointing down.	
Dorsiflexion	This term refers to bending the foot at the ankle joint so that the foot is pointing up.	
Circumduction	This is the circular movement of a part of the body as in doing 'windmills' with the arms. Circumduction can only occur at synovial joints.	

APPENDIX 2 THE APGAR TEST

The APGAR test, developed by Virginia Apgar in 1952, is a simple evaluation of a newborn baby's condition and covers five main areas:

- Activity and muscle tone
- Pulse (heart rate)
- Grimace response (medically known as 'reflex irritability')
- Appearance (skin colouration)
- Respiration (breathing rate and effort).

Each area is scored on a scale of 0 to 2 with 2 being the highest. When all areas are added together it gives a potential maximum score of 10 and potential minimum score of 0. A score of 7 or above after one minute is considered good. Anything less may mean that the baby requires

APGAR sign	2	1	0
Heart rate	Normal (above 100 bpm)	Below 100 bpm	Absent (no pulse)
Breathing (rate and effort)	Normal rate and effort, good cry	Slow or irregular breathing, weak cry	Absent (no breathing)
Grimace (responsiveness)	Pulls away, sneezes, or coughs with stimulation	Facial movement only (grimace) with stimulation	Absent (no response to stimulation)
Activity (muscle tone)	Active, spontaneous movement	Arms and legs flexed with little movement	No movement, 'floppy' tone
Appearance (skin colour)	Normal colour all over (hands and feet are pink)	Normal colour (but hands and feet are bluish)	Bluish-gray or pale all over

immediate medical attention. A score of less than 7 after five minutes usually means that the baby will require further medical care. It must be pointed out, however, that the test is not meant to predict long-term health, as a low APGAR score is normal for some newborn babies.

APPENDIX 3

For PARmed screening forms please visit: www.csep.ca/cmfiles/publications/parq/parmed-xpreg.pdf

APPENDIX 4 BODY MASS INDEX (BMI)

One of the easiest methods (but not the most accurate) to indirectly measure body fat percentage is body mass index (BMI). It is a very common method which simply divides a person's weight by their height squared (height multiplied by height).

BMI formula:
BMI = Weight (kg)/Height squared (m²)

According to the National Institute for Health and Clinical Excellence (NICE) a BMI below 25 is considered to be low risk whereas a BMI of 25–29.9 is classed as overweight and 30 or above is classed as obese (see table below).

However BMI does not take into account body composition (fat and lean tissue), so an individual with high muscle mass may have a BMI in the obese category but would not be at the same risk as an individual with a similar BMI due to excess body fat. BMI may also be inaccurate in women who are pregnant or breastfeeding or frail adults.

Classification	BMI (kg/m²)
Underweight	Less than 18.5
Healthy weight	18.5–24.9
Overweight	25–29.9
Obesity class I	30–34.9
Obesity class II	35–39.9
Obesity class III	40 or more

GLOSSARY

Absolute contraindications Conditions or circumstances where exercise is contraindicated

Adaptation Change due to repeated stimuli such as resistance training

Aerobic In the presence of oxygen

Aerobic fitness The ability to deliver oxygen to the working muscles and use it during exercise

Afterbirth A collective term for the placenta, umbilical cord and amniotic sac/membranes, usually delivered a few minutes or hours after the baby

Agility A rapid whole-body movement with change of velocity or direction in response to a stimulus

Agonist Refers to a muscle or muscle group responsible for the main action

Air embolism An air bubble that becomes trapped in a blood vessel

Alpha fetoprotein (AFP) A protein produced by the foetus, AFP testing may be done to check the foetus for certain conditions such as spina bifida or liver disorders

Alveoli Air sac in the lungs

Amniocentesis A process involving withdrawal of a sample of amniotic fluid for the purpose of testing for chromosomal abnormalities and other conditions

Amnion The membrane in which the foetus develops

Amniotic fluid The fluid that surrounds the foetus in the uterus

Anaerobic In the absence of oxygen

Anaerobic capacity The total amount of energy that can be produced anaerobically during a bout of exercise

Anaerobic fitness The ability to perform maximal intensity exercise

Anaerobic power The maximal rate at which energy can be produced

Anaerobic threshold The point at which the energy demand of the exercise being carried out can no longer be met by the aerobic system

Anaemia Reduced levels of haemoglobin in the blood

Antagonist Refers to a muscle or muscle group responsible for opposing the main action

Apgar test Assessment of baby immediately after birth using the Apgar score

Aponeurosis A fibrous sheet of tissue to which muscles attach instead of to tendons. Abdominal aponeurosis connects abdominal muscles to the linea alba (see below)

Areola Area of pigmentation surrounding the nipple

Arrhythmia Deviation from normal heartbeat

Anterior superior iliac spine (ASIS) Often called the 'hip bones'

Asthma Type of obstructive lung disease

Atrium Chamber in the heart which receives blood from blood vessels

Blood pressure The force of the blood on the artery walls

Body mass index (BMI) An individual's body weight divided by the square of their height

Bradycardia Low resting heart rate

Braxton Hicks contractions 'Practice' contractions occurring in pregnancy, usually becoming stronger towards term

Breech presentation Where the foetus is lying feet or bottom down. This occurs in approximately 4 per cent of pregnancies

Calorie The amount of energy needed to increase the temperature of 1g of water by 1°C

Cardiac output The amount of blood pumped out of each ventricle per minute

Cardiovascular Relating to the heart and associated vessels

Cardiovascular disease Disease of the heart (and related vessels)

Carpal tunnel syndrome (CTS) Compression of the medial nerve in the wrist leading to tingling or numbness in the thumb, index and middle fingers.

Cell Basic structural and functional unit of life

Centre of gravity The point at which the body can be balanced

Cerclage A procedure where an incompetent cervix is sewn shut to avoid opening under pressure of pregnancy

Cholesterol A fat-like steroid used to form cell membranes

Chorionic villus sampling This involves a sample of placental cells being removed and tested for genetic defects

Collagen The key component of all connective tissue

Colostrum Fluid breast secretions occurring in late pregnancy and after delivery; also called 'first milk'

Conception Fertilisation of egg signalling the start of pregnancy

Congenital Term used to describe a condition that was present at birth

Contraction Electrical stimulation of muscle to shorten muscle fibres

Corpus iuteum The outer covering of ovarian follicle

Dehydration Water loss from a state of normal amounts of body water

Delayed onset muscle soreness (DOMS) Perceptions of post-exercise soreness

Developmental stretch A stretch held long enough to induce physical structure development to increase flexibility

Diaphragm Muscle used for breathing

Diastasis recti The separation of the linea alba following pregnancy

Diastolic The time between the ventricle contractions when they are filling

Dilation/dilatation The enlargement or widening of the cervix

Dizygotic twins Fraternal or non-identical twins

Doming A bulge occurring in the abdomen when the rectus abdominis is contracted if diastasis recti is present

Down's Syndrome A condition resulting from chromosomal abnormality

Dyslipidaemia Abnormal amount of lipids in the blood

Dyspnoea Shortness of breath

Ectopic pregnancy The implantation of a fertilised egg outside the uterus

Elasticity The ability to resist deformation and return to the original shape

Emphysema Destruction of the surface of the alveoli

Energy The capacity to do work

Endocrine system An integrated system of organs, glands and tissues that involve the release of extracellular signalling molecules known as hormones

Endometrium The lining of the uterine wall

Enzymes Proteins that can speed up chemical reactions

Epidural A type of anaesthesia used during labour/birth

Episiotomy An incision/cut of the perineum performed to facilitate childbirth

Expected delivery date (EDD) The anticipated date of delivery of the baby

Extension Movement at a joint in which the joint angle increases

Extrinsic motivation The task leads to a reward

Fallopian tube A tube connecting the ovary to the uterus

Fascia Type of connective tissue

Fast-twitch Type of muscle fibre associated with strength and speed

Flexibility The available range of motion around a specific joint

Flexion Movement at a joint in which the joint angle decreases

Foetus The developing baby in the uterus

Forceps Specially designed tongs used to assist birth

Fundus The top of the uterus. The fundal height is a measurement taken from the top of the pubic bone to the fundus and is used to estimate the growth of the foetus

Genetics A broad term relating to the science of genes, inheritance and heredity

Gestation The period of pregnancy

Gestational diabetes (GD) Impaired glucose tolerance or diabetes occurring during pregnancy

Gestational hypertension See pregnancy-induced hypertension (PIH)

Gland A group of cells that release hormones

Gravity Force of attraction caused by the earth

Haemorrhoids Varicose veins occurring in the anus

Haemoglobin Part of a red blood cell that carries oxygen or carbon dioxide

Heart rate (HR) The number of heart beats per minute (bpm)

Histamine A chemical in the body that has the effect of widening the airways

Homeostasis When the systems of the body are working optimally and within set limits

Hormone A chemical messenger in the body

Human chorionic gonadotropin (HCG) Hormone produced in pregnancy, maintains production of progesterone

Hyperemesis/hyperemesis gravidarum (HG) Severe or extreme nausea and/or vomiting during pregnancy

Hyperglycaemia High levels of blood glucose

Hyperlipidaemia High levels of fat in the blood

Hypertension High blood pressure

Hypertrophy Enlargement of an organ such as muscle

Hypoglycaemia Low levels of blood glucose

Hypotension Low blood pressure

Hypothermia A body temperature of below 35°C

Hypoxia Reduced oxygen supply to tissues

Incompetent cervix When the cervix is unable to remain closed during pregnancy; can increase risk of second trimester miscarriage

Induction When labour is started artificially

Insulin A hormone secreted by the pancreas, involved in the regulation of blood sugar levels

Intensity A measurement of the difficulty level or 'hardness' of the exercise

Internal rotation Rotation of a part of the body towards the midpoint

Intrauterine growth restriction (IUGR) Where the foetus does not grow in line with expected potential; also called 'small for dates'

Intrinsic motivation The task itself brings about the reward

In utero Inside the uterus

In vitro fertilisation (IVF) The process by which an egg is fertilised outside the body then transplanted into the uterus

Kegel exercises Exercises designed to tone the pelvic floor muscles

Ketones Chemicals in the body regarded as toxins

Ketosis A state where raised levels of ketones are present in the body

Kyphosis Curvature of the thoracic spine

Labour The term given to the process of delivery of baby and afterbirth from the uterus

Lactation The secretion of milk from the breasts

Ligament Tissue in the body that connects bone to bone, used for support

Lightening When the baby moves down into the pelvis in preparation for birth, also called 'dropping' and 'engaging'

Linea alba A band of tendon occurring at the aponeurosis of the abdominal muscles

Linea negra A dark line that develops along the linea alba during pregnancy

Lipid The overall term used to describe any fat-soluble molecule

Last menstrual period (LMP) Used to date the pregnancy

Lordosis Excessive primary curve of the lumbar spine

Lumen The channel within a vessel or tube

Macrosomia An abnormally large foetus

Mass The quantity of matter a body contains

Mastitis An inflammation of the breast often occurring while breastfeeding

Maximum heart rate (HR$_{max}$) The highest heart rate an individual can safely achieve through exercise stress

Metabolic equivalent (MET) A method of expressing energy expenditure

Metabolic rate The amount of energy expended at a given time

Metabolic syndrome A combination of abdominal obesity, hypertension, dyslipidaemia and impaired fasting glucose

Miscarriage Loss of the foetus before 20 weeks of pregnancy. Most common in weeks 8–12; also known as 'spontaneous miscarriage' or 'spontaneous abortion'

Monozygotic twins Identical twins, produced by the fertilisation of one egg

Multiple gestation A pregnancy with more than one foetus – twins, triplets, etc.

Muscular endurance The ability of a muscle or muscle group to perform repeated contractions against a resistance over a period of time

Muscular strength The maximum amount of force a muscle or muscle group can generate

Neural Relating to the nervous system

Neuromuscular Relating to the muscular and associated nervous system

Nipple Protruding structure in the middle of the breast, surrounded by the areola

Noradrenaline A stress hormone (also known as norepinephrine)

Obesity The percentage body fat at which the risk of disease to the individual is increased

Obstructive lung disease A condition/s where damage to the lungs or airways cause difficulty with expiration

Oestrogen Steroid hormone key to female sexual development, responsible for growth of foetus and breasts in pregnancy

Omphalocele Term used to describe an umbilical hernia

Osteoarthritis Inflammation due to erosion of bone surfaces

Osteoporosis A condition of reduced bone density

Ovary The female reproductive organ that is responsible for production of eggs and hormones

Ovulation Release of mature egg (ovum) from an ovary

Oxytocin A hormone that stimulates contractions in labour and milk production after birth

Physical activity readiness questionnaire (PAR-Q) A self-screening tool which can be used by anybody embarking on a fitness training programme

Pancreas Organ in the body that secretes insulin

Perceived exertion A subjective measurement of exercise intensity

Perineum The area between the vagina and the anus

Pica Craving or eating of non-food substances such as charcoal, paper, etc.

Placenta An uterine organ which attaches the embryo/foetus to the uterus and which provides nutrients and eliminates waste from the foetus

Placental abruption A condition where bleeding from the placenta leads to detachment of the placenta from the wall of the uterus. May be associated with hypertension and pre-eclampsia; also called 'abruptio placentae'

Placenta praevia A condition where the placenta is lying (fully or partly) over the lower part of the uterus

Plasma Major fluid component of blood in which blood cells are suspended

Platelets Clotting cells in the blood

Power The product of force and velocity: Power = Work (Force x Distance) ÷ Time

Pregnancy-induced hypertension (PIH) The development of raised blood pressure during pregnancy; also known as 'gestational hypertension'

Presyncope A state of dizziness and/or weakness often preceding a faint

Preterm Relates to birth or rupture of membranes before 37 weeks

Progesterone A steroid hormone that prepares the endometrium for pregnancy and relaxes smooth muscle tissue during pregnancy

Prolactin Hormone responsible for stimulating milk production after delivery and stimulation of progesterone

Prone Lying on the front

Proprioception Sense of position in space

Proprioceptor A sensory nerve ending that monitors position of the body

Proprioceptive neuromuscular facilitation (PNF) This is a type of stretching

Residual volume The volume of gas remaining in the lungs at the end of a maximal expiration

Resting heart rate (RHR) The heart rate at resting levels measured in beats per minute (bpm)

Restrictive lung disease A condition/s where the lungs cannot fully expand thus restricting inspiration

Repetition maximum (RM) The maximum amount of weight one can lift in a given exercise for one repetition

Round ligaments The ligaments that support the uterus

Rupture of membranes The breaking of the amniotic sac, often referred to as 'waters breaking' and an indication that labour is started/will start soon

Scoliosis Twisting of the spine

Screening A process used to determine health status

Serotonin A chemical that can induce vasoconstriction; also has an effect on mood state

Slow-twitch Type of muscle fibre associated with endurance

Smooth muscle Muscle found in the walls of hollow organs that is not under voluntary control

Stability A body's resistance to the disturbance of equilibrium

Stillbirth When there are no signs of life in a foetus after 24 weeks

Stretching The method or technique used to influence the joint range of motion

Stretch marks Areas of stretched skin due to hormones and/or expanding abdomen

Stroke A rapid onset disturbance to brain function, the effects of which last more than 24 hours

Stroke volume The amount of blood ejected from one ventricle per heartbeat

Supine Lying on the back

Syncope Loss of consciousness or fainting, often due to a fall in blood pressure

Synergist a muscle or mucles that work together with the prime mover to assist or stabilise movement

Systolic Maximum pressure on the artery walls during contraction of the left ventricle

Tendon Connective tissue that surrounds muscle fibres

Termination A medically directed miscarriage that can be legally carried out before 24 weeks; also referred to as 'abortion'

Testosterone A steroid hormone that is responsible for muscle growth

Thermoreceptor A sensory nerve ending, responds to changes in temperature

Thermoregulation The regulation of temperature using various systems within the body

Tidal volume The volume of air that is inhaled or exhaled with each breath

Tissue A collection of cells with a physiological function

Total lung capacity (TLC) The maximum volume to which the lungs can be expanded with the maximum possible inspiratory effort

Transversus abdominis (TA) Muscle of the core, involved in forced expiration

Umbilical cord A cord-like tissue strand connecting the foetus and placenta

Uterus Pear-shaped pelvic organ, site of implantation of fertilised egg (ovum)

Vasoconstriction Narrowing of the lumen of blood vessels

Vasodilation Increase in size of lumen of blood vessels

Vein A vessel that carries blood back to the heart

Ventricle A chamber in the heart that receives blood from the atrium

Vestibular Balance information sent to the brain as a result of the mechanism of the inner ear

Voluntary As a result of conscious thought

VO$_2$ Symbol for oxygen consumption

VO$_2$max Symbol for maximal oxygen consumption, the maximum amount of oxygen that can be delivered to the working muscles

Watts A unit of power

Waist to hip ratio (WHR) The ratio of the circumference of the waist to that of the hips which is an indicator of the health of a person

Womb A term for the uterus

REFERENCES

American College of Obstetricians & Gynecologists (1994) 'ACOG Technical Bulletin No.189: Exercise during pregnancy and the postpartum period'. *International Journal of Gynecology and Obstetrics* 45: 65–70

American College of Obstetricians & Gynecologists (2002) 'ACOG Committee Opinion No.267: Exercise during pregnancy and the postpartum period'. *Obstetrics and Gynecology*, 99: 171–173

American College of Obstetricians & Gynecologists (2003) *Exercise during pregnancy. ACOG patient education*. Washington, DC: ACOG

American Congress of Obstetricians & Gynecologists (2003) *Getting in shape after your baby is born. ACOG patient education*. Washington, DC: ACOG

American College of Sports Medicine (2009) *ACSM's Guidelines for exercise testing and prescription* (8th edition). London: Lippincott Williams & Wilkins

American Psychiatric Association (2000) *The diagnostic and statistical manual of mental disorders* (4th edition) Text revision. Washington, DC: APA

Artal, R., O'Toole, M. & White, S. (2003) 'Guidelines of the American College of Obstetrician and Gynecologists for exercise during pregnancy and the postpartum period'. *British Journal of Sports Medicine*, 37: 6–12

Artal, R., Romen, Y., Paul, R. & Wiswell, R. (1984) 'Foetal bradycardia induced by maternal exercise'. *Lancet*, 2: 258–260

Avery, N.D., Stocking, K.D., Tranmer, J.E., Davies, G.A. & Wolfe, L.A. (1999) 'Fetal responses to maternal strength and conditioning exercises in late gestation'. *Canadian Journal of Applied Physiology*, 24: 362–376

Baddeley, S. (1999) *Health related fitness during pregnancy*. UK: Mark Allen Publishing

Baechle, T.R. & Earle, R.W. (2008) *Essentials of strength training and conditioning* (3rd edition). National Strength and Conditioning Association. Champaign, Illinois: Human Kinetics

Baker, C. (2006) *Pregnancy and Fitness*. London: A & C Black

Bauer, P.W., Broman, C.L. & Pivarnik J.M. (2004) 'Exercise and pregnancy survey for health care providers'. *Medicine and Science in Sports and Exercise* 36(5): Abstract. S113

Barakat, R., Stirling, J., Zakynthinaki, M. & Alejandro, L. (2008) 'Acute maternal exercise during the third trimester of pregnancy, influence on foetal heart rate'. *Revista Internacional de Ciencias del Deporte*, 13(4): 33–43

Bowden, J., Manning, V. (Eds). (2006) *Health promotion in midwifery*. London: Hodder Education

Ceysens, G., Rouiller, D. & Boulvain, M. (2006) 'Exercise for diabetic pregnant women'. *Cochrane Database of Systematic Reviews*, Issue 3: CD004225

Clapp, J.F., Little, K. & Capeless, E. (1993)

'Foetal heart rate response to sustained recreational exercise'. *American Journal of Obstetrics and Gynecology*, 168: 198–206

Clapp, J.F. (2000) 'Exercise during pregnancy. A clinical update'. *Clinical Sports Medicine*, 19: 273–286

Clapp, J.F., Kim, H., Burcio, B., Schmidt, S., Petry, K. & Lopez, B. (2002) 'Continuing regular exercise during pregnancy: effect of exercise volume on fetoplacental growth'. *American Journal of Obstetrics and Gynecology*, 186: 142–147

Clarke, P.E. & Gross, H. (2004) 'Women's behaviour, beliefs and information sources about physical exercise in pregnancy'. *Midwifery*, 20: 133–141

Collins, C., Curet, L. & Mullin, J. (1983) 'Maternal and fetal responses to a maternal aerobic exercise program'. *American Journal of Obstetrics and Gynecology*, 145: 702–707

Da Costa, D., Rippen, N., Dritsa, M. & Ring, A. (2003) 'Self-reported leisure-time physical activity during pregnancy and relationship to psychological well-being'. *Journal of Psychosomatic Obstetrics and Gynaecology*, 24: 111–119

Dale, E., Mullimax, K. & Bryan, D. (1982) 'Exercise during pregnancy: Effects on the fetus'. *Canadian Journal of Applied Sport Science*, 7(2): 98–103

Davies, G.A., Wolfe, L.A., Mottola, M.F. & MacKinnon, C. (2003) 'Joint SOGC/CSEP clinical practice guideline: Exercise in pregnancy and the postpartum period'. *Journal of Obstetrics and Gynaecology Canada*, 25: 516–529

Dempsey, J.C., Sorensen, T.K., Williams, M.A. Lee, I.M., Miller, R.S., Dashow, E.E. & Luthy, D.A. (2004) 'Prospective study of gestational diabetes mellitus risk in relation to maternal recreational physical activity before and during pregnancy'. *American Journal of Epidemiology*, 159: 663–670

Dempsey, J.C., Butler, C.L. & Williams, M.A. (2005) 'No need for a pregnant pause: physical activity may reduce the occurrence of gestational diabetes mellitus and pre-eclampsia'. *Exercise and Sport Sciences Reviews*, 33(3): 141–149

DiFiore, J. (2003) *The Complete Guide to Postnatal Fitness*, London: A & C Black.

Evans, J., Heron, J., Francomb, H., Oke, S. & Golding, J. (2001) 'Cohort study of depressed mood during pregnancy and after childbirth'. *British Medical Journal*, 323: 257–260

Evenson, K.R., Savitz, D.A. & Huston, S.L. (2004) 'Leisure-time physical activity among pregnant women in the US'. *Paediatric and Perinatal Epidemiology*, 118: 4000–4007

Flaxman, S.M. & Sherman, P.W. (2000) 'Morning sickness: a mechanism for protecting mother and embryo'. *The Quarterly Review of Biology*, 75(2): 113–148

Goodwin, A., Astbury, J. & McMeeken, J. (2000) 'Body image and psychological well-being in pregnancy. A comparison of exercisers and non-exercisers'. *Australian and New Zealand Journal of Obstetrics and Gynaecology*, 40: 422–447

Gorski, J. (1985) 'Exercise during pregnancy: maternal and foetal responses. A brief review'. *Medicine and Science in Sports and Exercise*, 17(4): 407–416

Guyton, A.C. & Hall, J.E. (2005) *Textbook of Medical Physiology* (11th edition). Philadelphia, PA: Saunders

Hemant, K., Satpathy, K.F., Fleming, A., Frey, D., Barsoom, M. & Satpathy, C. (2008) 'Maternal obesity and pregnancy'. *Postgraduate Medicine*, 120: 3

Hopkins, S.A., Baldi, J.C., Cutfield, W.S., McCowan, L. & Hofman, P.L. (2010) 'Exercise training in pregnancy reduces offspring size without changes in maternal insulin sensitivity'. *Journal of Clinical Endocrinology and Metabolism*, 95(5): 2080–2088

Institute of Medicine, Committee to re-examine IOM pregnancy. Rasmussen, K.M., & Yaktine, A.L. (Eds) (2009) *Weight gain during pregnancy, re-examining the guidelines*. Washington, DC: National Academy Press

Jovanovic, L., Kessler, A. & Peterson, C. (1985) 'Human maternal and foetal response to graded exercise'. *Journal of Applied Physiology*, 58: 1719–1722

Kalra, H., Tandon, R., Trivedi, J.K. & Janca, A. (2005) 'Pregnancy-induced obsessive compulsive disorder: A case report'. *Annals of General Psychiatry*, 4(1): 1

Kardel, K.R. & Kase, T. (1998) 'Training in pregnant women: effects on fetal development and birth'. *American Journal of Obstetrics and Gynecology*, 178: 280–286

Krans, E.E., Gearhart, J.G., Dubbert, P.M., Klar, P.M., Miller, A.L. & Replogle, W.H. (2005) 'Pregnant women's beliefs and influences regarding exercise during pregnancy'. *Journal of the Mississippi State Medical Association*, 46(3): 67–73

Lee, A.M., Lam, S.K., Sze Mun Lau, S.M., Chong, C.S.Y., Chui, H.W. & Fong, D.Y.T. (2007) 'Prevalence, course, and risk factors for antenatal anxiety and depression'. *Obstetrics and Gynaecology*, 110(5): 1102–1112

Leiferman, J.A. & Evenson, K.R. (2003) 'The effect of regular leisure physical activity on birth outcomes'. *Maternal and Child Health Journal*, 7: 59–64

Leigh, B. & Milgron, J. (2008) 'Risk factors for antenatal depression, postnatal depression and parenting stress'. *BMC Psychiatry*, 8: 24

Lokey, E.A., Tran, Z.V., Wells, C.L., Myers, B.C. & Tran, A.C. (1991) 'Effects of physical exercise on pregnancy outcomes: A meta-analytic review'. *Medicine and Science in Sports and Exercise*, 23: 1234–1239

Lynch, A.M., McDonald, S., Magann, E.F., Evans, S.F., Choy, P.L., Dawson, B., Blanksby, B.A. & Newnham, J.P. (2003) 'Effectiveness and safety of a structured swimming program in previously sedentary women during pregnancy'. *Journal of Maternal-Fetal and Neonatal Medicine*, 114(3): 163–169

MacPhail, A., Davies, G.A., Victory, R. & Wolfe, L.A. (2000) 'Maximal exercise testing in late gestation: Fetal responses'. *Obstetrics and Gynecology*, 96: 565–570

Manders, M., Sonder, G., Mulder, E. & Visser, G. (1997) 'The effects of maternal exercise on foetal heart rate and movement patterns'. *Early Human Development*, 48(3): 237–247

McMurray, R., Mottola, M., Wolfe, L., Artal, R., Millar, L. & Pivarnik, J. (1993) 'Recent advances in understanding maternal and foetal responses to exercise'. *Medicine and Science in Sports and Exercise*, 25(12): 1305–1321

Medforth, J., Battersby, S., Evans, M., Marsh, B. & Walker, A. (2006) *Oxford Handbook of Midwifery*. Oxford: Oxford University Press

Mørkved, S. (2007) 'Pelvic floor muscle training during pregnancy and after delivery'. *Current Women's Health Reviews*, 3(1): 55–62

Morris, S.N. & Johnson, N.R. (2005) 'Exercise during pregnancy: A critical appraisal of the literature'. *Journal of Reproductive Medicine*, 50(3): 181–188

National Institute for Health and Clinical Excellence (2008) *Obesity: The prevention, identification, assessment and management of overweight and obesity in adults and children (NICE public health guidance CG43).* London: NICE

O'Connor, P.J., Poudevigne, M.S., Cress, M.E., Motl, R.W. & Clapp, J.F. III. (1990) 'Safety and efficacy of supervised strength training adopted in pregnancy'. *Journal of Physical Activity and Health*, 8(3)

O'Neill, M., Cooper, B., Mills, C., Boyce, E. & Hunyor, S. (1992) 'Accuracy of Borg's rating of perceived exertion in the prediction of heart rates during pregnancy'. *British Journal of Sports Medicine*, 26(2): 121–124

Owe, K.M., Nystad, W. & Bø, K. (2009) 'Association between regular exercise and excessive newborn birth weight'. *Obstetrics and Gynecology*, 114(4): 770–776

Paisley, T.S., Joy, E.A. & Price, R.J. (2003) 'Exercise during pregnancy: A practical approach'. *Current Sports Medicine Reports*, 2: 325–330

Petersen, A.M., Leet, T.L. & Brownson, R.C. (2005) 'Correlates of physical activity among pregnant women in the United States'. *Medicine and Science in Sports and Exercise*, 37: 1748–1753

Pivarnik, J.M., Chambliss, H.O., Clapp, J.F., Dugan, S.A., Hatch, M.C., Lovelady, C.A., Mottola, M.F. & Williams, M.A. (2006) 'Impact of physical activity during pregnancy and postpartum on chronic disease risk'. *Medicine and Science in Sports and Exercise*, 38: 989–1006

Price, S. (2007) *Mental Health in Pregnancy and Childbirth.* London: Elsevier

Poudevigne, M.S. & O'Connor, P.J. (2006) 'A review of physical activity patterns in pregnant women and their relationship to psychological health'. *Sports Medicine*, 36: 19–38

Rafla, N. & Cook, J. (1999) 'The effect of maternal exercise on foetal heart rate'. *Journal of Obstetrics and Gynecology*, 19(4): 381–384

Rankin, J. (2002) *Effects of antenatal exercise on psychological wellbeing, pregnancy and birth outcome.* London: Whurr Publishers

Riemann, M. & Kanstrup-Hansen, L. (2000) 'Effects on the foetus of exercise in pregnancy'. *Scandinavian Journal of Medicine Science and Sports*, 10(1): 12–19

Sorensen, T.K., Williams, M.A., Lee, I.M., Dashow, E.E., Thompson, M.L. & Luthy, D.A. (2003) 'Recreational physical activity during pregnancy and risk of preeclampsia'. *Hypertension*, 41: 1273–1280

Stevenson, L. (1997) 'Exercise in pregnancy. Part 2: Recommendations for individuals'. *Canadian Family Physician*, 43: 107–111

Van Doorn, M., Lotgering, F., Struijk, P., Jan Pool, B. & Wallenburg, H. (1992) 'Maternal and foetal cardiovascular responses to strenuous bicycle exercise'. *American Journal of Obstetrics and Gynecology*, 166: 854–859

Wolfe, L. 'A Pregnancy'. In Skinner J.S. (Ed.) (2005) *Exercise testing and exercise prescription for special cases*, Baltimore, MA: Lippincott Williams & Wilkins

Wolfe, L. & Mottola, M. (1993) 'Aerobic exercise in pregnancy: An update'. *Canadian Journal of Applied Physiology*, 18: 119–147

Wolfe, L. & Weissgerber, T. (2003) 'Clinical physiology of exercise in pregnancy: A literature review'. *Canadian Journal of Obstetrics and Gynecology*, 25(6): 451–453

Wolfe, L., Brenner, I. & Mottola, M. (1994) 'Maternal exercise, foetal well-being and pregnancy outcome'. *Exercise and Sport Science Reviews*, 22: 145–194

Yeo, S., Steele, N.M., Chang, M.C., Leclaire, S.M., Ronis, D.L. & Hayashi, R. (2000) 'Effect of exercise on blood pressure in pregnant women with a high risk of gestational hypertensive disorders'. *Journal of Reproductive Medicine*, 45(4): 293–298

Zeanah, M. & Schlosser, S.P. (1993) 'Adherence to ACOG guidelines on exercise during pregnancy: Effect on pregnancy outcome'. *Journal of Obstetric, Gynecologic, and Neonatal Nursing*, 22: 329–335

FURTHER READING

Anthony, L., *Pre- and Post-Natal Fitness* (American Council of Exercise, 2002)

Baker, C., *Pregnancy and Fitness* (A&C Black, 2006)

Butler, J. M., *Fit and Pregnant* (Acorn Publishing, 1996)

Clapp, J.F., *Exercising through your Pregnancy* (Addicus Books, 2002)

DiFiore, J., *Postnatal Fitness* (A&C Black, 2003)

Hanlon, T.W., *Fit for Two* (Human Kinetics Campaign, 1995)

Mackin, D., *Getting back into Shape* (Dorling Kindersley, 2003)

USEFUL WEBSITES

American Congress of Obstetricians and Gynecologists (ACOG) www.acog.org

American College of Sports Medicine (ACSM) www.acsm.org

Association of Chartered Physiotherapists for Women's Health (ACPWH) www.acpwh.org.uk

Canadian Society for Exercise Physiology (CSEP) www.csep.ca

Royal College of Midwives www.rcm.org.uk

Royal College of Obstetricians and Gynaecologists (RCOG) www.rcog.org.uk

National Institute of Clinical Health and Excellence (NICE) www.nice.org

Net Doctor www.netdoctor.co.uk/health_advice/facts/pregnantexercise

NHS Choices www.nhs.uk/Planners/pregnancy-careplanner/Pages/PregnancyHome.aspx

The Association of Chartered Physiotherapists in Women's Health www.womensphysio.com

The National Childbirth Trust www.nct-online.org

World Health Organization (WHO) www.who.int

ANSWER SECTION

TRY THIS! See page 4.

Calculate the expected delivery date from the following LMP dates:

24 January = 31 October 2012
16 August 2007 = 23 May 2008
5 April 2008 = 12 January 2009

TRY THIS! See page 11.

Write down as many physiological changes that you can think of that occur in the body as a result of pregnancy. To help you, think hormonal, cardiovascular, respiratory, metabolic, gastrointestinal, postural and body temperature.

Table 3.1	Physiological changes during pregnancy
Changes	**Description**
Hormonal changes:	
• Relaxin release.	This is released from ovaries up to about 12–14 weeks when it is then released from the placenta. It can loosen ligaments postnatally for up to 6 months.
• Oestrogen release.	The levels tend to remain high throughout pregnancy as it promotes foetal growth, causes breast enlargement and stimulates colostrum production.
• Progesterone release.	The levels are high throughout pregnancy as it relaxes smooth muscle, stabilises blood pressure and stimulates colostrum. Greater insulin sensitivity to glucose can occur due to hormone level increase.

Changes	Description
Thermoregulation changes:	
• Mother's core temperature goes up.	Temp can increase by 0.6°C at the start and remain elevated for about 20 weeks.
• Pregnant glow.	Some areas of skin become hotter by up to 2–6°C.
• Increase in heat loss.	In early pregnancy heat dissipation is increased by up to 30% and in late pregnancy by up to 70% due to increased body mass.
• Quicker sweating.	Because the blood flow to skin increases and the breathing rate elevates, both increasing heat loss.
Cardiovascular changes:	
• Blood volume increases.	The volume of blood in the body can increase by as much as 30–40% to help supply oxygen to the foetus.
• Red blood cell mass increases.	Red blood cells can also increase by as much as 20–30% in order to supply oxygen to the foetus.
• Blood vessel walls dilate.	The size of the blood vessels increases to allow greater blood flow which results in something known as vascular underfill.
• Resting heart rate rises.	RHR can rise by as much as 10–15bpm.
• Cardiac output increases.	The amount of blood pumped out of the heart every minute can increase by about 30%.
• The left ventricle enlarges.	The chamber in the heart that pumps blood to the body can enlarge by about 20%.
• Blood flow to the skin increases.	This occurs to help cool the body.
Respiratory changes:	
• Increased ventilation rate and depth.	This just means that breathing increases and the amount of air taken in and out (tidal volume) increases by about 40–50%.
• The brain is more sensitive to levels of carbon dioxide.	This is partly responsible for the increase in breathing rate.
• Decreased residual volume.	The amount of 'spare' space in the lungs decreases.
• Increased oxygen consumption.	The amount of oxygen that is used up from the air increases by up to about 30%.
• Hyperventilation can occur.	This can be common at about 12 weeks due to the release of the hormone progesterone.

Changes	Description
Metabolic adaptations:	
• Resting metabolic rate increases.	The amount of energy used in the body at rest can increase by up to 20%.
• Symptoms of mild diabetes.	This is due to a delayed insulin response.
• Carbohydrate energy supplies preferentially used by foetus.	There is a high usage of carbohydrate by the foetus.
• Maternal blood sugar levels dip.	This happens about every 6–8 hours due to the usage by the foetus.
Gastrointestinal changes:	
• Relaxation of smooth muscle tissue.	Progesterone relaxes smooth muscle tissue which can lead to slower digestion and increased incidence of constipation, haemorrhoids (piles) and indigestion. Acid reflux can also occur which can lead to vomiting and dehydration.
Postural and musculoskeletal changes:	
• Centre of gravity disturbance.	During the growth of the baby the centre of gravity of the mother changes, which affects not only posture but also the stress on certain muscles that have to deal with this posture change.
• Diastasis recti.	As a result of the abdomen swelling (due to the foetus) the tendon band that keeps the rectus abdominis muscle in place can split to allow for growth. This is called diastasis recti.
• Ligament relaxation	Because of the increase in the hormone relaxin, the pubic symphysis (bones in the pubic region) can become less stable and cause pregnancy-related pelvic girdle pain (previously known as symphysis pubis dysfunction), and in some cases separate (known as diastasis symphysis pubis) which can cause severe pelvic girdle pain.

TRY THIS! See page 50.

Think of as many benefits to mother and baby that can be gained by exercising before and during pregnancy. This could be either physiological or psychological.

Benefits of physical activity

Mother:

1st trimester	2nd trimester	3rd trimester	Postnatal
Reduce or alleviate symptoms of pregnancy.	Increased energy levels and reserve.	Increased self-esteem.	Leaner baby.
Social aspects.	Improved digestion.	Better posture.	Quicker return to pre-pregnancy weight and fitness.
Maintain bone density throughout.	Reduced weight gain (fat).	Improved sleep.	Reduced bone loss.
Decreased risk of diabetes.	Reduced back pain.	More energy.	Reduced risk of depression.
	Enhanced maternal well-being.	Shorter and easier labour.	

Baby:

Foetuses of exercising women tolerate labour better than the foetuses of non-exercising women.

Foetal stress levels are lower in women who exercised throughout pregnancy (at 50% of their preconception level) compared to well conditioned athletes who discontinued exercise before the end of their first trimester.

Babies born to exercising mothers tend to be of similar dimensions (length and head circumference) but have less fat on them than babies born to non-exercising mothers.

TRY THIS! See page 54.

See if you can write down any guidelines that you think might be related to exercise during pregnancy.

Physical activity guidelines

General guidelines: If women are reasonably active prior to becoming pregnant and are generally healthy, then there should be no problems in continuing recommended activity throughout the pregnancy. However, if the individual was sedentary prior to becoming pregnant it is recommended that only low intensity activity should be undertaken.

RCOG, ACOG and ACSM guidelines:

	Aerobic Training	Strength Training
MODE	Walking, cycling and water based activities are good for this condition.	Continue as normal if already active. If not, slow progression from body weight to machines/free weights.
INTENSITY	• RPE level 10–14. • 60–80% HRmax.	• Avoid heavy loads. • Overload by increasing repetitions.
DURATION	• 5–45 minutes per session. • Increase by 2 mins per week but only between 13 and 28 weeks.	• Perform 1 to 3 sets of 15–20RM. • 1–2 minutes rest between exercises.
FREQUENCY	Active person: • 3–4 per week up to week 14. • 3–5 per week up to week 28. • 3 per week after week 28. Non-active person: • None before week 13. • 3 per week between 13 and 36 weeks. • 1–2 per week after week 36.	• 2–3 sessions per week. • Encourage other forms of exercise. • Decrease weight and sets and increase recovery time as pregnancy progresses.
PRECAUTION	• Avoid high impact activities and excessive repetition. • Watch for signs of overheating.	• If no experience prior to pregnancy, do not start. • Avoid overstretching and overhead lifts.

TRY THIS! See page 67.

Set some appropriate process goals for a pregnant woman based on the following aims:

Process goals during pregnancy

Aim	Process goal
I want to get back in pre-pregnancy clothes as soon as possible after my pregnancy.	Be aware that weight will increase during pregnancy and for a period afterwards. Therefore try to maintain any exercise programme as well as possible and only increase the intensity, duration or frequency in the postnatal period and only when it is considered best to do so. Be flexible with the time period.
I want to keep exercising throughout my pregnancy.	This should only be a goal if there were pre-natal exercise levels. Levels should not be increased and can also decline due to sickness associated with pregnancy. Therefore goals that are based on exercising whenever is appropriate should be set.
I do not want to get too round shouldered as a result of the pregnancy.	Aim to include resistance type exercises that focus on muscles of the back such as erector spinae, trapezius, rhomboids, latissimus dorsi and posterior deltoids. If the exerciser is not used to this type of exercise then start at a very low intensity.
I want to keep running at my current pace throughout pregnancy.	This is just not possible or appropriate. Many factors will influence this therefore reduce the target to just exercising as frequently as possible throughout pregnancy, but focussing on a session-by-session goal as opposed to an overall goal.

TRY THIS! See page 74.

Say the following phrase out loud placing the emphasis on the word in italics. Note what you feel is the key message that comes across with each phrase.

Change of word emphasis	
I said you were probably right	This suggests placing importance on the instructor saying the statement to infer that they should always be listened to as an authoritative source.
I *said* you were probably right	This is almost like an 'I told you so' scenario in which the client might not have believed the instructor was giving them credit but tries to re-iterate it after the event.
I said *you* were probably right	A possible miscommunication in which the instructor is reinforcing the message that the client is right.
I said you were *probably* right	The instructor is acknowledging the input from the client but is still inferring that they might not be right.

TRY THIS! See page 90.

For each sport or type of exercise below place a tick in the box or boxes that a component of fitness relates to.

Components of fitness for sports and exercise activities

	Cardio	Muscular Strength	Muscular Endurance	Flexibility	Balance	Speed	Agility	Power
Aerobics	✔		✔					
Aqua	✔		✔					
Ballroom dancing	✔		✔		✔			
Bowling		✔	✔	✔	✔			
Cycling	✔		✔					
Darts					✔			
Gymnastics		✔	✔	✔	✔			✔
High jump		✔			✔		✔	✔
Resistance training		✔	✔					
Running	✔		✔					
Swimming	✔		✔	✔				✔
Tai Chi			✔	✔	✔			
Tennis	✔		✔	✔	✔	✔	✔	✔
Walking	✔		✔					
Yoga			✔	✔	✔			

TRY THIS! See page 97.

Identify a location in the body for each muscle. Write down where you think each muscle attaches and what function it will have in pregnancy.

Muscle locations and their function during pregnancy

Rectus abdominis	Lower ribs to pelvis	Support uterus
Triceps	Shoulder blade to back of upper arm	Helps in any pushing movement
Bicep	Front of shoulder to front of lower arm	Main muscle responsible for lifting
Pectoral	Sternum across to inside of upper arm	Help support increase in breast weight
Trapezius	Running each side of the upper spine across to the shoulder blades in a diamond shape	Stabilises the shoulder blades to help posture
Latissimus dorsi	Runs up each side of the back under the upper arm	Helps when lifting in a bent over posture
Deltoids	Around the shoulders into the outside of the upper arm	Helps to stabilise the shoulder joints
Quadriceps	Front of the thigh from the knee running over the front of the pelvis	Contributes to leg strength to cope with the weight increase
Hamstrings	Back of the thigh from the knee running over the back of the pelvis	Contributes to leg strength to cope with the weight increase
Calf	From the heel running up the back of the lower leg to the knee	When walking is one of the main contributors to help blood circulation
Tibialis anterior	Front of the lower leg from the ankle to just below the knee	Helps to cope with the change in centre of gravity when walking
Hip abductors	Outside of the hip crossing the pelvis	Contributes to hip stability when walking
Hip adductors	Inside of the thigh running down to the knee	Contributes to hip stability when walking
Gluteus maximus	Posterior (bottom) area covering the back of the pelvis	Contributes to pelvic stability
Hip flexors	Front of the upper thigh crossing the pelvis	Contributes to hip stability when walking
Transversus abdominis	Like a wide belt going around the waist	Helps to stabilise the spine
Erector spinae	Narrow muscles running the length of the spine (either side)	Keeps good posture in the upper body

TRY THIS See page 102.

Place a tick in the box that is relevant to each sport in terms of importance of flexibilty.

Flexibility requirements for various sports and events			
	Low	**Medium**	**High**
Aerobics		✔	
Dancing		✔	
Netball		✔	
Running/jogging		✔	
Darts	✔		
Snooker		✔	
Cycling		✔	
Badminton		✔	
Tennis		✔	
Archery	✔		
Gymnastics			✔
Martial arts			✔

Try this! See page 114

Identify the suitability of the following types of session during pregnancy.

Suitability of exercise classes during pregnancy

Type	Yes	No	Cautions	Alternative
ETM (Exercise to music)	✔		Low impact and low intensity classes are suitable in the first trimester, however after 16 weeks supine lying is to be avoided and intensity will need to be reduced.	Dedicated antenatal class after 16 weeks or Aqua
Gym	✔		Studio resistance classes if already experienced but reducing the intensity through the pregnancy.	Body conditioning
Aqua	✔		Pool temperature may need to be adjusted to avoid cooling down or overheating.	ETM
Yoga	✔		Only specific antenatal yoga sessions with an appropriately trained instructor are suitable, other types such as hot yoga and dynamic yoga are not suitable.	Pilates or Tai Chi
Pilates	✔		After week 16 of pregnancy, any exercise that places stress on the rectus abdominis or oblique muscles should be discontinued to minimise the risk of diastasis recti.	Yoga or Tai Chi
Outdoor		✔	As this tends to be circuit based it is not recommended for newcomers to exercise. Regular circuit goers can continue as long as they reduce intensity at CV stations and weight at MSE stations.	ETM and Body Conditioning
Combat classes		✔	Combat or martial arts sessions are generally high intensity and high impact so are not suitable during pregnancy. Additionally, the joints may work through a larger range, and be affected by momentum and impact, none of which are suitable during pregnancy. A further consideration is that it is hard to maintain good pelvic alignment for some of the moves.	ETM or Aqua
Group indoor cycling	✔		Only suitable for those experienced in this type of class and with a low-risk pregnancy due to the intensity of the session. Specific antenatal indoor cycling classes are available and these would be more appropriate than mainstream classes.	ETM or Aqua

INDEX